FINDING A
JOYFUL LIFE
IN THE
HEART OF PAIN

FINDING A JOYFUL LIFE IN THE HEART OF PAIN

D A R L E N E   C O H E N

S H A M B H A L A

Boston & London

2000

Shambhala Publications, Inc.
Horticultural Hall
300 Massachusetts Avenue
Boston, Massachusetts 02115
www.shambhala.com

"Message to a Monk Who Scribbles Verse" by Ikkyu from
Essential Zen by Kazuaki Tanahashi. Copyright © 1994 by
Kazuaki Tanahashi and David Schneider. Reprinted by
permission of HarperCollins Publishers, Inc. Selections of
Zen Master Dogen from *Moon in a Dewdrop: Writings of Zen
Master Dogen,* edited by Kazuaki Tanahashi. Reprinted by
permission of North Point Press, a division of Farrar,
Straus & Giroux.

9   8   7   6   5   4   3   2   1

First Edition
Printed in the United States of America

⊗ This edition is printed on acid-free paper that meets the
American National Standards Institute Z39.48 Standard.

Distributed in the United States by Random House, Inc.,
and in Canada by Random House of Canada Ltd

Library of Congress Cataloging-in-Publication Data

Cohen, Darlene.
    Finding a joyful life in the heart of pain / Darlene
Cohen.—1st ed.
        p.   cm.
    Includes bibliographical references.
    ISBN 1-57062-467-4 (alk. paper)
    1. Conduct of life. I. Title.

BF637.C5 C635   2000
158.1—dc21   99-053191

This book arose out of my need to express my relief and joy at having had the support and companionship of world-class teachers and friends throughout a tremendous ordeal, my life. I have come to realize that my anguish, terrible though it is to bear, is not very different from other people's. It is mundane. I would like to dedicate this book to the many people who looked deeply into their own suffering, found their own delight, and told me their stories.

~

MESSAGE TO A MONK WHO SCRIBBLES VERSE

Pain and bliss, love and hate, are like a body and its shadow;
Cold and warm, joy and anger, you and your condition,
Delight in singing verse is a road to Hell,
But at Hell's gate—peach blossoms, plum blossoms.

—IKKYU

~

CONTENTS

❧ ❧

CONTENTS

ACKNOWLEDGMENTS

I am very grateful to Tony Patchell, my husband, who brought me to Zen practice in the first place, whose forbearance of my self-absorption is rather heroic, and whose garbage mind has penetrated and dissipated my cloud of abstraction over and over. To you, Tony, I owe my heart and intimacies of an unmentionable nature without number.

To Michael Wenger, who reeled me in when I was setting up standards of my own because I was convinced I could never be part of a vigorous Zen community again or teach zazen. He said "This is twentieth-century America. You can teach anything you want." It is Michael who has since taught me everything I wanted to know and stuff I lacked the sense to want to know.

To Elizabeth Sawyer, who not only grabs me by the psychic lapels and shakes me conscious from time to time but who has made of her own suffering a means of penetration into the nature of reality.

To Daya Goldschlag, whose insistence on integrity and dignity in all her relationships has transformed my own ability to appreciate and seek intimacy with other people.

To Richard Baker, who took me on at the beginning, taught me earnestly and sincerely the way of Suzuki-roshi, and then sacrificed his own life at Zen Center in order that I might shift my focus to my own way.

To Sherrie Echols, who plunged me into the world of workshop-giving and generously shared her expertise. She always pushed the envelope, always insisted on acknowledging what was there. I sometimes clung to her psychic skirts, terrified, while she orchestrated intense group dynamics replete with tears and joy. The inquiry that resulted in this book would have been impossible without her initial inspiration and guidance.

To my other teachers along the way: Reb Anderson, Blanche Hartman, Shunyru Suzuki, Dainin Katagiri, Linda Ruth Cutts, Teah Strozer, Yvonne Rand, Ethan Patchell, Meir Schneider, Joseph and Winifred Cohen, David Chadwick. Thank you. You all persisted past the point of reason.

I am also indebted to Michael Katz, my agent, who generously and skillfully helped me shape my ideas and experiences into a cogent book.

My editor at Shambhala Publications, Emily Hilburn Sell, not only answered all my questions with speed and clarity but is also good-humored and kind. She is ultimately responsible for this book as well, in that she originally showed interest in its being published after editing my chapter in *Being Bodies*. Emily, thank you, thank you.

I must also thank Walker & Company, New York, publisher of my first book, *Arthritis: Stop Suffering, Start Moving,* for its very generous permission to use parts of that book in this one. Jacqueline Johnson, my editor there, has been especially helpful and responsive to my requests.

PART ONE

✧

SUFFERING

THE PROBLEM

Caught under the Ever-Turning Wheel of Grasping and Aversion

❧ ❧

CATHERINE was a highly successful financial consultant in downtown San Francisco, a young woman thriving in a man's world, reveling in all the rewards that business acumen can bring: luxurious condo, designer wardrobe, everything but disability insurance. After her car accident, she found herself living with and financially dependent on her mother again, just as she had been as a child.

Ricardo played soccer every weekend before he herniated a disk at work; soccer games had been the center of his social world, and his prowess the cornerstone of his identity. He had been married only a year, but he could no longer make love to his energetic, vivacious wife. Forced into the role of househusband while his wife supported them, he was depressed and humiliated.

Two years after her adored sister died of cancer, Emily seemed to be functioning just fine. She worked, had a family life, pursued hobbies. But suddenly and unpredictably, she still burst into tears and cried effusively. It was as if her sister's death had opened up some old, deep wound that would never heal.

Melanie was the overworked office manager of a small construction firm owned by other members of her family. She found that the scheduling, correspondence, billing, and payroll responsibilities demanded much more than one full-time employee. To keep up with her job, she worked into the night and on weekends. Not only did she worry constantly about the work that was not getting done, but she was also beginning to bitterly resent her uncle's refusal to hire an assistant for her. Her waking hours were now defined by stress and anxiety so severe that she was developing physical symptoms.

❧

MANY OF US in the course of living our everyday lives endure terrible suffering: grief or anxiety or depression or physical pain that won't go away. I think of this kind of suffering as "mundane" anguish, affliction rendered bearable only because it's part of our everyday lives, like drawing breath or doing the dishes. If we ever got relief from it, we would suddenly apprehend how dreadful it actually is. Depression and anxiety can be so overwhelming that they are as crippling as a disease or an injury. When we are chronically depressed or anxious, we become so trapped in the habit of thinking terrifying or destructive thoughts that we simply cannot function with a clear mind. Our own feelings are no longer our touchstone for reality.

Others of us may have contracted a physically debilitating disease or been injured in such a way that our lives and those of our family have been changed forever. It doesn't even take a specific loss to experience mundane anguish. We humans suffer just because everything changes all the time. Having once achieved some goal, we can't rest on our laurels. All of life's circumstances are dynamic, ever evolving into something else. We clutch at security in vain.

I myself have had rheumatoid arthritis, a very painful and crippling condition, for twenty years, and the stress of the disease—the fear of the future and the despair at what has been lost already—is often worse than the physical pain that I am suffering at any particular moment. When the disease first struck me, I was forced to stay in bed. I lost forty pounds. I couldn't dress myself, hold the phone receiver, or get up from the toilet unassisted. I was completely overcome by unremitting pain, fatigue, and despair. In four months of deterioration, I lost everything that meant anything to me: reliance on a strong, young body; my achievements and the sense of self-worth they brought me; my pleasure in being a sexually attractive woman; my identity as a mother; and my ability to do the required practices and sustain myself in the community in which I lived as a student of Zen meditation. I became isolated from everyone I knew by my pain and fear and ultimately even by the consuming effort I had to make to do any little thing—like get up from a chair, pick up a cup of tea.

How do we live through unbearable situations like a catastrophic disease without being destroyed? How do we deal with the mundane anguish of our everyday lives? How do we continue to live under crushing stress? And even further, how do we not just get through these things but have rich, full, and worthwhile lives that we actually want to live—under any circumstances?

It might at first seem easiest to ignore mundane anguish, but if this attitude hardens into a way of life, then chronic anxiety, loss of sleep, or physical symptoms may appear and force us to face the fact that something has to change. This may mean that if so much of our lives involves stress and pain and suffering, we have to actually face and acknowledge our suffering in order to live our lives fully. We may need to become familiar with the thoughts and feelings that define our suffering to us, notice how we as individuals perceive our own suffering and the suffering of those around us, and catch the exact moment when we decide it's too much and automatically tune out. If we don't acknowledge our pain, we usually don't feel our pleasure strongly, either. Life takes on a zombielike tenor.

One of the saddest stories a client ever told me came from an elderly woman who sought my help in dealing with her arthritis. With her husband, she had worked long and hard for some years in order to afford their dream vacation, a cruise to the Caribbean islands. She and her husband had never allowed themselves any pleasures in their ordinary lives because they were saving everything for their vacation of a lifetime. When they finally had enough money to take their monthlong trip, they were beside themselves with excitement. The time that they had been looking forward to for so long had at last arrived. After they returned, I asked my client how the trip had gone. Shaking her head, she replied:

> It was disappointing. We were given an itinerary at the beginning, listing all the activities, mealtimes, and stops we would make. It seemed so exciting at first. We did everything, ate all the meals, and stopped at all the different islands to shop and sightsee. But we were always looking at the itinerary to see what was coming next. Somehow that seemed more exciting than what we were doing now. What happened was that we were always looking forward to the next event. Finally, the trip was over, and it was like it never happened.

She and her husband had spent so many years ignoring the life that was under their noses and available to them, looking forward to a life that was to come someday, that when someday arrived, they couldn't rise out of their habit pattern to meet it. They had been focused on the future for so long, they couldn't refocus on the present. It receded like the rest of their lives into habit and routine. Her plaintive story brought tears to the eyes of listeners when she told it again later at a meditation retreat. And hopefully, it struck fear into everybody's heart. Because if we continually choose to blank out our feelings about our mundane suffering and always keep our eyes on the future, how different are our lives from those of this woman and her husband?

What is it that you must have in order to live a rich, fulfilling life, relatively free of dead or "numbed-out" spots? I don't think you have to have the perfect body, buffed up from the gym, or the Right Man/Woman waiting for you at night, freedom from economic pressures, extensive training in spiritual disciplines, or even a meaningful job—thank God!—to be deeply involved in your life. You don't even have to change the circumstances of your life to enrich it vastly. I think you can engage your life and sink your roots deeply into every situation in the midst of high stress, terrible pain and suffering, physical disability, or paralyzing anxiety.

You only need to break the bad mental habit of living your life on automatic pilot and cultivate the necessary skills to actually be present enough to live the moments of your life, however miserable or boring your life situations might seem when you compare them to your fantasies. You need to learn how to be alive for all of your life, to be present as much as you can, not to pick and choose the moments that you think are worthwhile to be alive and then be numb for the rest. Because just as a muscle gets weak from disuse, so your ability to be present in your life fades if you don't practice it. As Thich Nhat Hanh points out in an early meditation manual called "The Miracle of Being Awake":

> There are two ways to wash the dishes: the first is to wash the dishes in order to have clean dishes and the second is to wash the dishes in order to wash the dishes. If we wash them only to get them out of the way with an eye to the cup of tea after, we are not alive during the time we are washing the dishes. In fact we are completely incapable of realizing the miracle of life while standing at the sink. If we can't wash the dishes, the chances are we won't be able to drink our tea either. We will only be thinking of other things, barely aware of the cup in our hands. Thus we are sucked away into the future, incapable of actually living one minute of life.

Our intelligence and dignity themselves are developed by our being alive for everything, including the mundane anguish of our lives. Just our awareness of our sensations, of our experience, with no object or idea in mind, is the practice of not preferring any particular state of mind. Intimacy with our activity and the objects around us connects us deeply to our lives. This connection—to the earth, our bodies, our sense impressions, our creative energies, our feelings, other people—is the only way I know of to alleviate suffering. To me, our awareness of these things without preference is a meditation that synchronizes body and mind. This synchronization, the experience of deep integrity, of being all of a piece, is a very deep healing. It is unconventional to value such a subtle experience. It is not encouraged in our culture. We're much more apt to strive to feel special, uniquely talented, particularly loved. It's extraordinary to be willing to live an ordinary life, to be fully alive for the laundry, to be present for the dishes. We overlook these everyday connections to our lives, waiting for the Big Event.

GRASPING AND AVERSION
THE EVER-TURNING WHEEL OF PAIN AND PLEASURE

If you're like me, your daily emotional life is like being tied to a wheel traveling over all different kinds of terrain, ranging from sun-spattered gardens to suffocating mud. You just keep going up and down, hour after hour. First of all, there's the basic mood I wake up with, which provides the background against which I'm going to interpret the events of the early morning. If that mood is energetic and expansive, I will be predisposed toward everything that happens; if that mood is sour or shaky, everything that happens will be an imposition on my consciousness, an ambush from an aggressive and demanding outer world.

That basic mood can be changed by anything that happens during the day. If I get a phone call from a good friend while I'm doing my morning exercises and we hang up having shared plenty of laughter, I'm ebullient as I dress. But then I put on a well-loved skirt and feel the snugness of the fit. I'm immediately upset by the reminder that I've put on some weight in the last few years. Even when I pull another, better-fitting, skirt out of the closet, I'm not cajoled. My self-disgust tape starts running: "I'm fat, I've lost my girlhood figure, and I'm just another stout matron, nobody special anymore." But then I manage to pull together an outfit, it's a good hair day, a little lipstick—and hey, the total effect isn't that bad. I begin to feel a little space in the diaphragm area; I've got some breathing room in there after all. The day could be salvaged.

The phone rings. It's a client canceling her arthritis therapy appointment with me. She didn't foresee she would have to study for an exam tomorrow instead of see me, though she was desperate when she made the appointment. For me, it's a buzz of irritation; I could have scheduled the desperate person who called yesterday. The breathing room I got from looking good vanishes. I voice my annoyance at the late notice she's given me, although it is within the twenty-four-hour safety zone. She's intimidated by my irritation, and her tone is appeasing. I don't allow myself to be completely appeased. We make a new appointment. I hang up annoyed with her, angry at my unreasonable reaction, and the day is dark again. My self-pity tape kicks in: "I'm unappreciated by my clients, who don't realize how much I do for them and how valuable my time is, blah blah blah."

The phone rings again. This time, it's a friend who leads a weekly meditation group. "My group enjoyed your talk so much the last time you came," he says with great enthusiasm. "I wonder if you'd come again and give a talk in two weeks." His ebullience penetrates my dark energy. My heart is lifted out of its self-pity, and another, more pleasant, tape starts running: "At last, my wisdom has been recognized. His group members will sit smiling back at me while I expound my own personal version of the dharma. I'll tell a few stories, we'll all laugh, they'll adore me, and I'll be happy." This is a good tape.

I enter the kitchen to make my morning tea with a broad smile on my face. I love my kitchen, with its handmade crockery and yellow walls. Every object has some meaning, some connection to a friend. I got married late in life, so I still have wedding gifts I use. I love kitchen utensils and the sounds they make while being used, running the water into the kettle, the clink of its bottom on the burner, the whoosh of the gas flame going on. Soon the aroma of my tea fills the room. Ah, life is good. I cut a peach and a banana into a bowl and turn to the refrigerator to get the yogurt to round out my delicious, nutritious breakfast. My eyes search the top shelf where it usually is, and a small twinge of fear tightens my chest—I don't see the yogurt. My eyes then go to the bottom shelf, their shifting movements a little more frantic, and then finally, disbelievingly, I understand: there's no yogurt! How can this be? Other family members have finished it off, not considering that I need nutrition more than any of them! I slam the door shut, angry, hurt, undone. There is the fruit glistening in the bowl. I can't even get my mind around any substitute, it's all so tragic! I leave the kitchen brokenhearted and start preparing the therapy room for my first client. It is barely 9:00 AM.

I spread the fresh, clean-smelling sheet, renew the pillowcase, straighten the room, and feel good again. I love this room even more than the kitchen. The sun streams in through the lace curtains; rainbow colors fleck the wall, refracted by the sun's rays bouncing off the crystal hanging in the window. When you lie down on the massage table, you see the clouds on the ceiling, painted by one of my clients in exchange for therapy. A Balinese angel spreads her wings out over the room from her place on high; artwork and poetry from clients fill the backs of the shelves behind my massage oils and cassette tapes. Who wouldn't feel glorious in this room dedicated to comfort and strewn with the objects of friendship and healing? I am such a lucky person, I reflect, my mood basking in the sunlight as well.

I feel even better after working with my client. She feels terrific, I feel responsible, we both commune our good feelings. She pulls on her socks and shoes, and I rewind the cassette tape I have made of movements for her to do at home. She leaves, and I am energetic and important and valuable in my world. It doesn't get better than this.

I play back a couple of messages that came in while I was working. The first one jolts me out of my self-satisfaction. A medical facility at which I've been teaching meditation for nearly a year is canceling my next seminar because it has decided to change its image. It's going to emphasize concrete career-building skills like taking apart car engines and stop offering "transformative" classes like stress reduction. My megatape starts running—not the one about how I personally am unappreciated but the one about how the whole world is too blind to realize that the kind of work I and other visionaries do is an indispensable contribution to everyone's sanity and well-being. Now I'm really upset! Having been hurled into a craving state of mind, I wander into the kitchen, make myself some toast, and eat the fruit I cut this morning without even tasting it. I glance at the clock on the microwave. It's not even noon and I've been all over the map: in heaven, in hell, in summer's bounteous garden, in winter's bleak landscape.

And this is my emotional life at its best, its most even. What I've just described is a "normal" morning in a regular, ordinary life, not one in which any crisis has taken place. My grandson got off to child care, my son and husband to their jobs; our home is still standing with all services working; our car is parked outside at the curb awaiting my use later in the day. It languishes securely in its parking place; no one has crashed into it during the night as has happened twice before. And despite my rheumatoid arthritis, I am not in great pain this morning. So my emotional life is playing itself out within the fairly constricted limits of an ordinary day. But even without a crisis, the highs and lows are pretty vivid.

I wouldn't have it any other way. I value all these feelings as life-affirming, as threads in the rich and complex tapestry of my ongoing daily life. I'm willing to be pulled along, to soar among the gods and plummet to the hard ground, although some part of me watches the whole process with disbelief, shaking its head in wonder at what it is to be alive.

What is human life about? I suspect the half day I described above is typical of most of us who continue to stay in touch with our feelings instead of obliterating them. We recoil from pain; we embrace pleasure. That's it in a nutshell. Can we find any neutral thoughts in our brains? We might locate a sensation or two that qualify as neutral, like yawning or having an object touch our skin that is neither irritating nor pleasant. But the overwhelming majority of our thoughts and impulses concern our relentless grasping after pleasure and avoidance of pain. We get trapped in that; most of us do without respite forever. The great stories of our civilization, all the tragedies ever written, the tales that come down to us through the ages have as their theme the quest for pleasure or the grief of loss. Any of our lives could be such a tale. It does not occur to most of us that we are virtual prisoners of our primal preferences, positive or negative, but we are.

I know not everyone is as willing as I to entertain these emotional characters inside me who seize my full attention, one after

the other, all day long. Many people find this unbearable, desta-
bilizing, exhausting, and they develop strategies to avoid strong
feeling. They're willing to sacrifice feeling altogether in order to
get rid of the bad feelings. Some people hold on desperately to
neutral territory. Stuff happens to them, but they just keep on as
if it hadn't. Their world is gray and undefined, comforting like
fog. The sun may not shine there, but neither are there hurri-
canes and tornadoes.

STRATEGIES FOR GETTING OFF THE WHEEL

Compulsive Busyness

Many people spend years developing a strategy to insulate themselves from feeling their feelings: they bury themselves in activity
the way a substance abuser buries herself in drink or drugs; no
matter how many things she races to do during the day, there's
always something more to be done. When there is a threat of
hurt or disappointment due to circumstances beyond her control, there's no time to feel it. The laundry has to be put in the
dryer; the kids have to be picked up; the report has to be finished; the car has to be washed. The overall feeling is unpleasant
enough, frantic, strangled, but she does manage to avoid the real
lows: the grief, the anger, the disillusionment.

I knew a woman who dealt with bad feelings in this way. After
years of feeling strangled and resentful of the fact that her kids
were growing up without her really noticing, she decided to try
to change her habit of busyness. She rearranged the priorities of
her daily life and dropped anything she thought was unnecessary
to her job and her roles as wife and mother. The first thing she
noticed was how depressed she felt. This amazed her. She had
thought she was going to feel relief and then happiness. Instead,
she started to see exactly why she had developed the habit of
busyness; in other words, she began to feel the old feelings of
hopelessness and despair she remembered from her youth. She
told me, "It's like mowing the lawn to be able to see all the wild-
flowers and instead seeing all the weeds!" I advised her to spend

some time every day looking at the weeds, examining their shape and color, studying them without interruption. She seemed startled by my suggestion but was intrigued. She had nothing to lose. In another few months, the weeds had parted. Not only had she discovered a bottom to her feelings of hopelessness and despair, but the nuances of these dreaded feelings gave some sort of subtle, agreeable flavor to her time with her children, like some perspective against which to appreciate the passage of time with them. I find this woman's account of penetrating her mundane anguish fascinating.

Always a Victim, Never a Vulnerable Person

Another strategy we use to deal with painful feelings is the victim stance: always blaming something outside ourselves for circumstances that are challenging or disagreeable. Many times we are right: there is some outside factor that has precipitated our misery, and we should voice our objections to the person or institution that disempowered us. But often, even after obtaining redress, we are still in a victim stance, this time over something else. We only feel comfortable when we're addressing some outside cause of our internal feelings of self-hatred. We can spend our lives this way and feel triumphant at each victory—or at the very least, righteously outraged at each defeat—but if we assume this particular stance at every turn in our lives, we continually feel disconnected from most situations and many people. No amount of personal success or adulation will fill our pit. We'll always walk alone, us and our outrage.

As a case in point, I know a successful novelist whose knee-jerk reaction to any unpleasantness is a lawsuit. No amount of personal success and admiration has persuaded her that anyone outside her very small circle of friends does not have as his or her goal her personal annihilation. Because she is so smart and clever, she has developed this worldview into an art form. Outside her strict writing hours, she spends considerable energy talking to lawyers and describing the wrongs done to her. I always considered this quirk of hers a mere pimple on the surface of her bril-

liant mind, until I noticed over the years how small her circle of
trusted intimates had gotten. Last year it consisted only of her
husband and one of her daughters. Because I have known and
admired her for so long, it feels funny to realize that she really
has become the archetypal "bitter old prune," the angry woman
who has narrowed her options so severely her world is bleak.

Addiction

Not only do we Americans flatten out the curve of emotional
volubility with our addictions to alcohol, food, and drugs, but our
habit pattern of avoiding pain by returning again and again to
the same favorite states of mind—to sex, excitement, crisis, compulsive work—also constitutes an addiction. As Robert Aitken
points out in *The Mind of Clover,* "Addiction . . . set[s] up a pattern of avoiding the low emotional places in life. The best therapy is the practice of acknowledging one's feelings and making
friends with them. Then they can be seen as truly transparent."
When thoughts are perceived as "transparent," it means that we
can see through them to their source: the ceaseless busyness of
our minds. Thoughts and feelings follow each other, one after
the other, in a constant, ever-changing flow. If we can be quiet
enough to watch this flow with curiosity rather than agitation, it
seems quite arbitrary to become disturbed or transported by any
particular one.

Yet this doesn't mean that if we see their transparency, we become indifferent to our thoughts and feelings. We continue to
have them, of course, but we have a choice about whether to
believe they are the only point of view to which we can subscribe.
Robert Aitken continues: "Feelings, whether of compassion or
irritation, should be welcomed because both are ourselves. The
tangerine I am eating is me. I clean this teapot with the kind of
attention I would have were I giving the baby Buddha or Jesus a
bath. Nothing should be treated more carefully than anything
else. In mindfulness, compassion, irritation, mustard green and
teapot are all sacred."

PLEASURE AND ADDICTION
A SLAVE IN THE REALM OF THE GODS

It's probably clear to everyone why we humans might reflexively avoid pain and discomfort, and thus why we would want to discontinue whatever behavior brings them on, but it's not so obvious what the downside is when we compulsively chase after pleasure. We all want to attain pleasure in some form or another. Some of us have simple needs: a full belly, a sexual partner, the esteem of our fellows. Some of us make it our life's work to achieve "peace of mind" or to experience something called "religious ecstasy." We hear these words a lot in connection with spiritual matters. And it may be that the possibility of ecstasy or serenity is what attracts many people to take up the rigors of meditation practices in the first place.

Most of us decide to begin a meditation practice when we're in the pain aspect of the pain-pleasure cycle. We're suffering in various ways, and it occurs to us that we suffer precisely because of our perceptions of things, that there's something wrong with those perceptions, and we want to escape our suffering into some more agreeable state of mind. So we begin to practice meditation in order to alter those defective perceptions and expand our knowledge of various states of mind. I came to meditation for this reason. When I first heard the Four Noble Truths of Buddhism—that life is suffering; that desire, in the form of grasping and aversion, is the cause of all suffering; that we can cease desire-based suffering; and here's how—I said, "That's for me!" I was absolutely thrilled that somebody had been doing research on this problem for thousands of years.

Even though it certainly feels better to experience pleasure than pain, and it therefore seems eminently reasonable to prefer it, in fact, chasing after pleasure doesn't deliver us from the clutches of misery. Often pleasure fails to relieve our depression or anxiety for more than a brief interlude, and the chase itself actually exacerbates them. We are all intelligent enough to manipulate our world to achieve pleasure, but we can't hold onto it once we get it, nor can we always get just the thing that we think would please us. Sometimes when we get what we want, it doesn't please us as we thought it would—or at all. "Be careful what you pray for," the wise woman counsels. The particular pleasure we want may be too hard to attain, like the admiration of a certain person. It may end too soon, like a sexual interlude. It may not be as thorough and distracting as we hoped, like a disappointing movie. Or if it does work for us—the sex was great and the movie good—then after a pleasant interval in which we are lolled into a sense of well-being, the pleasure ends, and we are plunged back into the world of suffering, all the worse for having been temporarily reassured. This is what usually happens when we finally get the desired job or marry the perfect mate. There is a honeymoon period, followed by a return to normal. In this way, pain and pleasure are constant companions.

Because we yearn so passionately to be forever happy, and we can imagine such a thing, we concoct the possibility of a sort of heaven, the complete elimination of pain and permanent state of pleasure. If we are very industrious, we get rich enough to acquire every physical comfort and surround ourselves with fawners. Or if our inclination is spiritual rather than material, and we finally figure out how to course in the realm of the gods, we have indeed achieved great bliss. Trungpa Rinpoche describes this state of mind in his book *Cutting Through Spiritual Materialism:* "We relax, dwell upon our achievements, shield out unpleasant thoughts. It's hypnotic, blissful, proud. Everything happens naturally, easily, automatically." We get parking places with no problem. We're always in the right line at the grocery store or the toll bridge. "When we are in the realm of the gods, whatever we hear is musical, whatever we see is colorful, whatever we feel is pleasant. We have achieved a kind of self-hypnosis, a natural state of concentration which blocks out of the mind everything that might be irritating or painful. It's a kind of trance state in which the empire of ego is completely extended to include everything; it has no boundaries."

Suddenly returning to real life from this hypnotic intoxication can sometimes be a terrible crash. The teenage daughter of a client of mine was arrested with three friends after the girls spent an afternoon on a shoplifting spree in a local mall. All were good students who had never been in trouble before. When my client arrived at the mall security office to pick up her daughter after the arrest, she found the child close to passing out with anxiety and self-loathing, a state of mind that continued for several days. She could not look at her mother or father, or even her little sister, without cringing with shame. What impressed both my client and me was that the girl seemed almost not to know the person who had done the stealing. "It was so amazing," she told her mother, her expression turning rapt even in describing what it had felt like to take things from so many stores without getting caught. "We felt after a while like we could do anything, have anything, even stuff we didn't care about, just because we were so special, such clever people." This is the realm of the gods. She said, "Now I can't even imagine what I was thinking then; it was like I was a different person. But it was great!"

While I was living at Green Gulch Farm, a Zen farming community, as a student of Zen, I popped into the realm of the gods for a fairly long period of time, a couple of months. I got good at keeping myself in there by means of concentration practices. It felt so wonderful to hang out there; everything went my way for a change. My perceptions were so stunningly clear, not only in organizing my activities but in relations with other people, that I assumed this state of mind was my reward after all that meditation. I had finally got enlightened like the meditation masters of ancient times. People actually started treating me differently after a time, more kindly and respectfully, perhaps because I had been so obnoxious before and now I was calmer, more open to other people's opinions. I felt very empathetic to everybody, even to the point of feeling sorry for them because they weren't as fortunate (advanced in their meditation practice) as I. Since I perceived the world generally as wondrous and beautiful, I wasn't nearly as irritable and impatient as had been my habit before.

After enjoying this state of mind for a few months, I began to feel trapped by it. Little by little, I started feeling lonely. Here I was, hanging out somewhere in the heavens with nobody to share it. And this heavenly state of mind left me feeling cut off from the more mundane concerns of my earthbound friends. I started noticing that there were subtle forms of suffering inherent in this blissful state of mind: worrying about its ending, being isolated, always being preoccupied with keeping my absorption going. Finally I really wanted to return to the ups and downs of ordinary life.

If you get attached to this state of mind, unwilling or unable to go on with your ordinary life, then it's as if you've fallen into some kind of pit. You lose your ability to relate to other people with their everyday concerns. Despite your wonderful state of mind, you're still experiencing some subtle suffering: you have to work to maintain this bliss, and you're worried you might get knocked out of it. But worst of all, perhaps even more than compulsive thinking or feeling sorry for yourself, constantly striving to maintain a blissful state of mind interferes with your ability to experience what's right in front of you.

A Zen student who had planned to do a one-day meditation retreat I was leading came up to me the day before the retreat and told me he couldn't sit with me after all because something had come up in his life. I was immediately concerned. I said I hoped nothing terrible had happened. He said, "Oh, no," and hastened to assure me that he was fine. Then he told me he couldn't meditate because he had gotten a promotion at work. He was very excited about getting more money and having more responsibility, and his mind was so agitated by these pleasant thoughts, he couldn't sit still. I consider this student mature enough to settle down during a day of meditating, or at least capable of observing every mental and bodily manifestation of his agitation if he had decided to join us for the retreat, but he chose not to. He didn't want to take the edge off his happy state of mind.

After I rejected the realm of the gods as a substitute for life, I was so relieved to be back that I started to be present during my ordinary, humdrum existence: doing the dishes, changing my baby's diaper, and arranging cheese and crackers on platters for guest conferences at Green Gulch Farm. The latter was a perfect returning-to-mundane-life task for me, even bordering on ironic, because it was an activity I'd been avoiding all my life. I grew up in the suburbs watching my mom arrange endless cheese plates for meetings of her women's groups, visits from relatives, holiday gatherings. They symbolized a meaningless life to me, and I swore I'd never have a lifestyle that involved arranging cheese on a platter. Here it was, my first job after leaving the realm of the gods. After I had been living my mundane life again for some weeks, I began to value it tremendously, as if it were a great privilege. I understood that my bliss state had been very narrow and that I had been living a very one-sided existence in the realm of the gods. I'd been going down a specific path, looking to neither the right nor the left, missing everything that was off to the sides. Ordinary life seemed now to be an explosion of experiences. I had a first-time-ever but deep appreciation for the rich complexity of human life.

Some people who explore "New Age" religions based on classical Eastern or Native American teachings interpret those teachings to mean that they're supposed to be happy and generous, upbeat and blissful, all the time. I used to meet people like that at Green Gulch Farm when I was working in the office on Sunday, which was visitors day. Relentlessly sunny and cheerful, they spoke of the spiritual path with great enthusiasm and were often generous enough to suppose that we at Green Gulch Farm were also sunny and cheerful as a result of our obviously arduous meditation practice. Outsiders sometimes find it difficult to relate to such devotees because they are nearly impervious. In their efforts to practice what they believe to be the teachings of their serene masters, they seem to bury any feelings of hesitation or gloom and so are inaccessible to those of us with "ordinary" consciousness. I'm embarrassed to admit that after talking to people like that for a while, I always wanted to kill something. I think I compulsively carry the shadow for people who choose not to do so.

Another stance commonly taken by students of the meditative arts is the impersonation of equanimity. Because Eastern religions emphasize the impermanence of all existence, practitioners of one of these systems might have the ideal of equanimity. If they've been practicing meditation for a while, they think they should be calm and serene all the time (or at least appear to be), as if the impermanence of every single thing and being and thought in the universe—even the universe it-self—were a situation they personally could live with. New students of meditation are very quiet, slow, and deliberate, seemingly imperturbable. They're commonly found at the cash registers of health food stores, especially when you're in a hurry. They manage to seem deliberate, careful, and oblivious all at once. This serenity lasts until some unfortunate event happens— everybody else at the retreat center eats all the dessert before they're able to get to the table, say—and then their equanimity is disturbed. So those who prefer a state of mind, or think religious practice itself is a particular state of mind, can find it very unsettling to lose their composure over petty things.

Traditionally, though, in Zen teaching, hanging out in a blissful state of concentration (*samadhi*) or even in what is popularly considered as the Zen cornerstone state of mind—equanimity—is regarded with suspicion. It's not lively enough. In *The Blue Cliff Record*, Hsueh Tou says in his verse: "Placidly walking along, he treads down the sound of the flowing stream; he has gone into the nest of entangling vines; The grasses grow thick; [He's fallen into equanimity]," implying that his equanimity has become a stance, a pit; thus trapped, he cannot experience the present moment.

At the end of that same verse, Hsueh Tou says, "Though you be clean and naked, bare and purified, totally without fault or worry, this is still not the ultimate. In the end, though, what is? Look carefully at this quote: 'I snap my fingers; how lamentable is *Shunyata*!'" *Shunyata* is a Sanskrit word for a pure mind free of troubling thought and concern. Thomas Cleary writes that in ancient China, snapping the fingers was used to ward off filth or taboo. Preferring the state of mind of equanimity is referred to in Chinese Zen as intoxication, considered one-sided, incomplete, and narrow-minded; hence, it is taboo. So in the Zen literature, equanimity *as a stance,* a habitual and preferred state of mind, is considered a pitfall of meditation practice, not an achievement.

But this idea of the permanent attainment of equanimity and bliss consciousness as the objects of meditation practice is very strong in our general culture. Sometimes when I am teaching meditation in hospitals or businesses as a way of coping with pain and stress and I refer to bliss as a distraction from concentration, similar to thinking about what you're going to do after the meditation class, people are quite startled. They think that the state of mind called bliss is the whole point of doing the meditation. What do I mean that it's a distraction? For their first session, I led a class of managers and lawyers in a guided meditation through the body—twenty minutes of following my steady, soothing voice instructing them to breathe into each body part and then breathe out. When I asked for comments and questions afterward, everyone was delighted with the experience, remarking, "So relaxing!" and "Very refreshing."

Then I began to instruct them in a slightly more demanding meditation: counting each breath from one to ten without my guidance. Usually when people do this for the first time, they notice with some amazement how active and distractible their minds are. When I asked for comments following this second meditation, one person immediately said that after the first few minutes, he had gone back to the previous meditation instead. I was surprised when several others agreed. "The first one was a great meditation!" they said. "Why do something difficult after you find something that works?" When I argued that the purpose of this class was to prepare them to face stressful situations with even-mindedness and awareness of choice while they were experiencing great stress, not to give them a bliss break once in a while, still some of them protested that the body meditation was enough for them. They were apparently resigned to getting very stressed out and upset during their workday as long as they could take time out in bliss states. Bliss states instead of coffee breaks. Despite such a beginning to this five-week class, several individuals did manage to become intrigued by a practice in which they learned not to prefer any state of mind but to live their whole lives to the fullest, welcoming all states of mind.

A very devoted and sincere Zen student in another meditation class told me that over the course of several weeks, he had at last achieved some calm in his life, which he attributed to meditation practice. He said, "I'm in bliss," meaning that he was in a good mood for an extended period of time, unusual for him. Because I know him as an ambivalent, anxious person who has trouble accepting his anxiety as the normal background for his activity, I was a little concerned when he told me he was in bliss. It seemed to be continuing for an unusually long time, and I didn't know how disappointed he would be when the blissful state of mind passed. Sure enough, a bad incident at work interfered with his bliss preoccupation, and he came out of his trance, making a conscious choice to abandon the trance in order to be present and take care of his social work client. I was not surprised when he told me he was actually relieved to be "back." I asked him, "Where is 'back'?" He said, "I'm back dealing with my problems, including all the different states of mind that come up." As I had done at Green Gulch Farm so many years ago, he began to appreciate ordinary states of mind that didn't seduce him or lash him to them, but rather allowed him to just let one thought follow another.

So from the point of view of living your life in a very rich, full way, open to everything that is going on, the states of mind of equanimity or bliss are not to be preferred any more than emotional upheaval or anger or being depressed or comforting a child. They're just two more states of mind, some of the thousands that visit us every minute, as natural to us as the air we breathe. At a meditation retreat in Spokane, a sitter asked me, "Where do all these thoughts come from?" When I said I thought that's just the inherent nature of the mind, a doctor in the group answered, "Think insulin and pancreas."

When we question whether our desperate flight from pain and frantic pursuit of pleasure is the way we want to spend the whole of our lives, then we begin to see the ironic and humorous quality of going around the wheel, of being raised up or cast down by life's constant variations, to laugh through the experience of struggle and chuckle at its futility. We go around on the karmic wheel over and over again. It's not so much a matter of getting off the wheel as of noticing our patterns. Very few of us discover that there might be an alternative to going through life this way, that there might be a radically liberating alternative predicated on both turning toward pain and intimately investigating pleasure. After I stopped devoting my mental energies to catapulting myself into the realm of the gods and began appreciating my ordinary life, I began to understand how someone could choose pleasure in a disinterested way and how that differs from addiction.

AT HELL'S GATE

Physical Pain as a Model for Suffering

ও ৵

I T has been said that pain is unavoidable, but suffering is optional. This implies that you can choose not to suffer. If you are running along a sandy white beach and turn your ankle, you feel physical pain. There may be inflammation and tenderness for a few days or weeks. Full-blown suffering, as distinguished from the pain, starts when you moan, "Oh, no. What if I've hurt myself badly enough that I'll never be able to run along the beach again? Without the joy of running freely like that, I'll be miserable!" And you worry for weeks about the meaning of every little twinge in your strained ankle. The pain is clear and sharp; it's physically unavoidable if you turn your ankle. The suffering is conceptualization about the pain, head stuff.

If your lover leaves you, you will feel the pain of loneliness and rejection. The loss of sex and companionship is surely one of life's worst trials. But extended suffering sets in if you pull the covers over your head and cry, "I knew I was unlovable! I'll never be loved again!" You deepen your anguish exponentially by interpreting this event as a confirmation of your worst insecurities.

It does seem certain that pain is clear, clean, and sharp—and unavoidable. Suffering is conceptualization about the pain, a step removed. But I question whether we really do have a choice about suffering. Rather than being just an annoying adjunct to pain that we could get rid of if we really tried, I think conceptualization about our pain may be how our minds inherently work.

When we leap out of our immediate experience of pain into ideas about our pain, it is true that we are a step removed from the experience of the pain, and it seems like needless aggravation to extend our pain by worrying about its consequences. But I think this is what human minds do: worry about the consequences. The upside is that if we are observant, we have a front-row seat to watch how an immediate experience inevitably deteriorates into a drawn-out pattern of stress. We can watch our mind leap into its dizzying spiral as an accompaniment to our pain, tearing through all the worst-case scenarios like a word processor on amphetamines, and we can smile, appreciating the intrinsic sniffing-puppy character of our minds. When we take our ideas about our suffering to be some kind of static truth and fail to see that our ideas can shift and change, then we are trapped.

I've often heard people in pain say, "I know it would be better if I could accept my pain, and I keep trying and trying, but I can't! I can't accept it; I hate it!"

I think many people have a skewed idea of what "accepting" pain is. If you have the idea that coping well should resemble serenity or equanimity, something like the proverbial "grace under fire," then you think you should resign yourself with a big cosmic grin, no matter what horrors are being visited upon you. Actually, "accepting" pain sounds to me too passive to accurately describe the process of successfully dealing with chronic pain. It fails to convey the tremendous energy and courage it takes to accept physical pain as part of your life. Truly accepting pain is not at all like passive resignation. Rather, it is active engagement with life in its most intimate sense. It is meeting, dancing with, raging at, turning toward. To accept your pain on this level, you must cultivate particular skills. After you have developed some proficiency, dealing with pain feels much more like an embrace, or the bond that forms between sparring partners, than like resignation.

What are the skills necessary for dealing with chronic pain, pain that you have day in and day out and probably will have for a long time? If you have chronic pain, your job is to (1) acknowledge that pain and its burden and (2) enrich your life exponentially. If, at any given moment, you are aware of ten different elements—for instance, the movement of your eyes as you focus on this page, your bottom on the chair, the sound of cars passing outside your room, the thought of the laundry you have to do, the hum of the air conditioner, the sliding of your glasses down your nose, an unpleasant memory of sharp back pain, cool air going into your nostrils, warm air going out, and throbbing pain in your hips—that's too much pain, one out of ten; that's unbearable pain that will dominate your life. But if, at that moment, you are aware of a hundred elements—not only the ten things you noticed before but more subtle things, like the animal presence of other people sitting quietly in the room, the shadow of the lamp against the wall, the brush of your hair against your ear, the pull of your clothes against your skin—and you have pain along with all those other things you are noticing, then your pain is one among a hundred elements of your consciousness at that moment, and that is pain you can live with. It's merely one among the multitude of sensations in your life.

This is coming at chronic pain from two angles: one is acknowledging it and understanding what it costs you in terms of suffering; the other is opening up your life, making it so rich that no pain can commandeer it. Before you lose your creative energy to depression and before you are disabled by somatic manifestations of your anxieties, you can begin to live with your suffering in such a way that life's frustrations and disappointments are part of the rich tapestry of living. In order to have such an attitude, you need to cultivate skills that enable you to be present for all of your life, not just the moments you prefer.

ACKNOWLEDGING YOUR PAIN AND SUFFERING

Acknowledging your suffering—exactly what it is costing you to live with your painful situation—is the first step on the path of penetration into the wellspring of your experience, and it holds tremendous potential for your liberation from depression and anxiety.

How do you learn to acknowledge your suffering? I think it lies in practicing respect for all your feelings. You must treat your anxiety, pain, or hatred gently, respectfully, not resisting it but living with it. When you do resist it, you need to treat that with respect, too. You must develop your capacity to appreciate each thing as it is now, while inundated with suffering. Nothing should be treated with more respect than anything else. When you are able to give all your feelings your full attention, without believing that one feeling is good and another bad (even if you think it is), then compassion, irritation, pain, hatred, and joy are all sacred.

An advantage of allowing yourself to feel your pain and restriction is that if you focus your attention on the sensations of your body, you get a tremendous amount of helpful information about that pain. Sensation is information about your body. Paying attention to your sensations—for example, under what circumstances you do and don't have pain—can give your brain the information it needs to formulate a solution. If your hips hurt sometimes but not all the time, you may begin to observe what makes them hurt and what relieves the pain. You try all postures—lying, sitting, and standing, and variations within those postures—and you begin to get an idea of exactly what influences the comfort of your hips. This is an information-gathering process, your observation of your sensations, and it is crucial to your being able to alleviate that pain.

This candid and inquisitive attitude toward feelings can extend to all the relationships you have with other people. Each relationship or encounter with another person requires your respect, your acknowledgment, though your response to each of them may be quite different. You can study your reaction to each one—your boss, your mother, the person hassling you on the street for spare change—to learn about yourself. If you give each encounter equal attention, then whatever other people present to you becomes an opportunity to study your own reactions, to discover the value judgments you make that cause you to cling to an idea or a person or turn away from someone in disgust. You can study the opinions that separate you from others, that keep you on the ever-turning wheel of grasping and aversion.

If you have some catastrophic change in your life, like disease or injury, one of the most difficult things facing you is letting go of the past—the easy, idyllic past—and focusing on the life you have now. It's easy to forget that even before the catastrophe, you didn't think of your life as easy. There was too much to do in too little time; you didn't see yourself as on top of things and in control, operating at peak efficiency. It is very difficult to have a strong, functional body displaced by a painful, helpless one. It shakes you to your very identity. In order to heal in this situation, you have to give up your past, to grieve your former body and then turn away, to learn to see your present body as real and your current life as demanding all the creativity and energy you can summon, maybe even more.

If we have lost the relative ease and mobility of the past, it may be hard to make a real commitment to this new life. There's a tendency to deny these new circumstances and wait for our old life to return. But in every moment, every day, every week we spend lamenting our lost life, we also have an opportunity to shift all our interest and creativity to this new life. Perhaps even more than in the past, our lives demand everything we can bring to them. The purpose of our lives may not be to produce something wonderful or to become rich or famous or renowned for wisdom; the purpose may just be to express our own sincerity doing completely whatever it is we do, immersing ourselves in the situation in which we find ourselves. When our way is very hard, we have an opportunity to use every flicker of our imaginative fire. This attitude gives us a tremendous sense of freedom and creativity. We feel as if we can imbue any situation with the richness of our own poetry.

After I was bedridden with rheumatoid arthritis, my mobility was so impaired that volunteers from the San Francisco Zen Center began cleaning my room, doing my laundry, and washing my hair. As my body got weaker and my pain greater, and I could no longer deny my situation, I realized that this is the life I have been given. This is the body I have to live the rest of my life with. Within my experience, this is my reality. Every day, I woke up and began to say, "What part of my body can I use today to do the things I have to do?" Strangely, I found relief in just being the suffering. Because I was so ill, nothing was demanded of me: no function, no performance, no self-sufficiency, no heroics. Just me living and breathing. This baseline life allowed me to live in a very simple, nondemanding way.

At first, my conscious life was all pain. Acknowledging the pain and its power eventually allowed me to explore my body fully and find there actually were experiences in my body besides the pain—here is pain, here is bending, here is breath, here is movement, here is sun warming, here is unbearable fire, here is tightness—something different wherever I looked. My life began to be filled with sensation. Not just pain but sensation of all kinds: children's voices outside my window; subtle changes in the shadows on the wall as the day passed; feeling my entire body when I turned over in bed, noticing the temperature differences in the various parts of my body, those inside and outside the covers; the contours of a familiar face. Rather than shrinking, my world was as intricate as ever, just on a much more subtle level. Because I was no longer goal-directed, sensation and feeling filled my consciousness. I kept telling myself this must be the world of babies and animals. Everything is fresh and fascinating.

Valuing these subtle experiences is very unconventional thinking; it is extraordinary to be willing to be involved with ordinary things, to be willing to live in the mundane. We don't have a lot of role models for this kind of attention in our society. Thus, we are very deeply touched when they appear to us. It is so moving when it does happen that it can inspire us for years. When I was first very sick, lying in bed, I happened to hear a recording of Mississippi Fred MacDowell's Delta blues music. He strums a guitar and sings in a rough voice. He plucks each string of his guitar as if it were his own heartstring he's vibrating to express his pain. When I heard him, I felt that if he could manage to touch a guitar string that way, I could try to live as sincerely as possible.

Injured or not, ill or not, we all have to face the deterioration of our bodies as we age. Most of us, the "temporarily abled," face it slowly rather than in one swift, unalterable blow. But if we live

long enough, we will know this suffering. We all have to give up
our bodies someday. The sick among us get in practice.

ENRICHING YOUR LIFE EXPONENTIALLY

If you are in great pain much of the time, it becomes absolutely
necessary that you create a life for yourself that you can not only
tolerate but love and enjoy. I am probably in more pain than
most of the people I know, yet I see my life as one of the most
pleasant ways of living currently available to human beings. I believe my life is enjoyable and satisfying because I take my pleasure
as seriously as my pain. And what I take most seriously is living
each moment of my life, to the extent that I am able to pay that
much attention. Another way to put this is that I try to do each
thing for its own sake, to experience every motion, every endeavor, every contact, for what it is. Washing the dishes is not just
about getting the dishes clean; it's about feeling the warm, soapy
water soothing my arthritic fingers and noticing the brief discomfort in my elbow joints when I lift a clean dish into the dish
drainer. Folding the laundry is an opportunity for smelling its
cleanness and luxuriating in the simple movements as a counter-
point to my complex life. There need be no better reason than
that I am alive and doing these activities. This is engagement that
arises out of a commitment to live as thoroughly as a human can.

How do we develop this appreciation of things just as they are,
the spacious and bountiful spirit of letting everything be, especially if we are sick and in pain? Our teachers tell us to look into
ordinary things. Thich Nhat Hanh says that combing our hair or
washing the dishes gets us in contact with reality. If we can do
this with full attention, there's no fantasy life going on, no goal
in mind, just our satisfying and complete activity. It works on a
purely somatic level as well. If we slowly turn a sore leg in bed or
feel our bones accept our weight, we are connected with real
stuff. For some of us, being sick is the first time we slow down
enough to notice our ordinary lives. Going to the bathroom and
rising from the toilet seat, hearing an airplane overhead or a dog

barking outside, feeling unaccountably appreciative of the flowers planted inside a mall, experiencing the sudden flash of irritation when a pen rolls off the table. Of course, these events happen to all of us all the time, sick or well, but usually we ignore them as mundane.

It turned out that the Zen meditation training I had had before falling ill was a great help in this way. I had been taught to study the objects of consciousness: feelings, perceptions, sensations, and thoughts. In long periods of meditation, I even had been able to watch my perceptions as they were being formed. This is, of course, the business of Zen meditation, to observe all these things. You simply focus your attention on what is happening now, the stream of your consciousness. There is no goal involved.

Before becoming so ill, I had trouble interrupting my discursive mind to make the observations necessary to begin a mindfulness practice. On a Sunday, I would vow to notice all my postural changes, determined to say to myself when I went from sitting to standing to lying: "Now I'm standing." "Now I'm lying." Then the next time I remembered—Thursday, say—I would suddenly cry, "Oh! I'm standing!" After becoming ill, I lived in a world of continual intrusive sensation because of my pain. I was highly motivated to make these observations. It was very much in my self-interest to notice what circumstances increased or decreased my pain and then to alter my pain level by manipulating those circumstances. Changing my posture was a dramatic event in my life. I needed to heed every little sensation in my legs and feet in order to go from sitting to standing.

I lived a half block from the San Francisco Zen Center and used to try to dine there once a week as a treat to myself. I would walk down the hill, which brought me to the bottom of a number of steps to the front door. Climbing the steps would be the second leg of a laborious journey. Sometimes I would make it all the way to the steps and be unable to go up them. So I would have to drag myself back up the hill to my apartment. I asked myself, "What is it about my walking that is so tiring?" What I called "walking" was the part of the step when my foot met the sidewalk. From the viewpoint of the joints, that is the most stressful component of walking. The joints get a rest when the foot is in the air, just before it strikes the pavement. I found that if I focused on the foot that was in the air instead of the foot that was striking the pavement, my stamina increased enormously. After making this observation, I never again failed to climb the steps to knock on the front door of Zen Center.

Struck that the focus of my attention could make that much difference in my physical ability, I began to search out the times my brain was clumping together many disparate motions into an idea that would prevent me from overcoming an obstacle. Then I concentrated on breaking down these aggregates of ideas into discrete units of smaller experience that I could master. Sick or well, we all do this all the time. We get into the idea of something, the clump, the heap, the pile, rather than the actual experience. Someone says, "I can't practice meditation because I haven't been able to get on my meditation cushion for three weeks," instead of just sitting still and being quiet when she can. When I haul out the carrots and cutting board during the arthritis workshops I give, everybody immediately groans, "I can't cut carrots with my arthritic hands!" But when they actually hold the knife in their hands, feeling its wooden handle and sharp, solid blade; and they touch the vulnerable flesh of the carrot on the cutting board; their wrists go up and down, up and down; and the orange cylinders of carrot begin to pile up on the board, they realize "I *can* cut carrots." Tears come to their eyes.

A woman who was in a wheelchair with a diagnosis of severe arthritis of the hips and spine came to me to learn how to spend some time out of the wheelchair, to walk around her house. I taught her many stretching and strengthening exercises so that her weak body could begin to support itself. For a long time, she did her exercises like taking medicine; she didn't actually live through them. I could tell that by her uninspired questions: how many of each exercise should she do, and what order should she do them in?

Then one session she greeted me with a big grin. She said with real delight in her voice, "I found out everything that happens to me is information about my body. Hurting or getting tired or not feeling like exercising. I'm noticing everything!" And I knew she had gone from mechanical movement into the timeless realm of sensation itself. The whole universe was her medicine.

So it's true that we can use meditation practice to achieve our health goals. We may even get rid of our disease or injury. But if we practice paying attention to our body mainly to get rid of our suffering or restore an ailing body to functioning rather than to express our life and our nature, it is a very narrow and vulnerable achievement. Just as a clay Buddha cannot go through the water or a wood Buddha cannot go through the fire, a goal-oriented healing practice cannot permeate deeply enough. We must penetrate our anguish and pain so thoroughly that illness and health lose their distinction, allowing us to just live our lives. Our relief from pain and our healing have to be given up again and again to set us free of the desire to be well. Otherwise, getting well is just another hindrance to us, another robber of the time we have to live, another idea that enslaves us, like any other achievement. Fortunately for our ultimate freedom, recurring illness is like a villain stomping on our fingertips as we cling desperately to our healthy, functioning bodies. Healing ourselves is like living our lives. It is not a preparation for anything else, nor a journey to another situation called wellness. It is its own self; it has its own value. It is each thing as it is. We live our lives to express our own sincerity, our own nature.

Ironically, my body was nearly immobile before I ever appreciated it. I had had a very strong, healthy body. Like a slave, it obeyed my commands. I rose at dawn to work in the fields of Green Gulch Farm, but I always thought, why am I so tired by dinnertime? I sat through hours of discomfort during daylong meditation retreats, but I always thought, why can't I sit with my legs crossed and my feet up on my thighs like real yogis? I used to run with the wind along the hills in Marin County, but I always thought, why can't I run farther? Then lying in bed unable to stand up alone, I thought, thank God for one part, *any* part, that still goes up and down. Even if your body is weak or painful, it's still your home; it's how you're manifesting this life. On the most

34   SUFFERING

basic existential level, your body is also your penetration into reality: it is the only way that you can experience the transparency and interconnections of all things.

COMFORT

Sometimes it just hurts too much; there's nothing to be done. You're out of energy; you're frustrated, angry, feeling sorry for yourself. You have no intention of "going into the feelings" or doing any self-exploration. You need a break. You need solace and comfort. You can either offer yourself some consolation by introducing another level of experience to those miserable feelings, which is like taking a crying child on your lap and stroking her hair, or you can distract yourself altogether, which is like handing that crying child a cookie.

Direct Comfort

Bodily movements and sensations that require a great deal of consciousness can be a highly effective form of consolation. While you are attending to your precise bodily sensations, you cannot be carried away by obsessive, destructive thoughts. Sensation and thought are neurologically incompatible at the same moment. You can only do one or the other.

In a dramatic example, a man who came to me as a client told me he wanted a relaxing massage. Because he was young and looked to be in excellent health, I asked him if he was in pain. He said no, he had no physical pain, but he was in such extreme anxiety over a situation facing him that he felt like taking his own life. As he spoke, I saw how troubled he was. He could barely look at me. He undressed for the massage with total disregard for his clothes, not noticing whether they landed on the chair when he tossed them. He was very preoccupied with his troubled thoughts. I worked on him for about twenty minutes, soothing his muscles and rubbing his head gently, but he didn't relax at all. He told me that even on my massage table, he couldn't stop thinking about his problem.

I went to the tape player and put on some really primal Delta blues music. The singer's pain was in his voice and in his strumming. My client listened for a few minutes, then began to weep. The guitar strings seemed to vibrate his chest. I could see it heave as Mississippi Fred plucked his guitar. Since he was so open to the sound, I encouraged him to feel the guitar strums as part of his body. Using the music, I took him into bodily sensation, including the sensations my massage was causing. I continued to massage his tight muscles, and I felt them relax at last.

At the end of an hour, he was a changed person. Even his voice was lower. He said, "You're absolutely right. You can't feel and think at exactly the same moment. Until now, I haven't had a second's relief since this problem appeared." I made a tape for him of gentle, comforting movements, such as lying on his back and moving his bent knees from side to side, rotating his lower arms around his elbows while turning his head from side to side, and so on. He came again the next day and the next until he felt he had it—"it" being the idea of substituting sensation for worry. This is a tremendously effective way to deal directly with anxious thoughts.

Another very good way to comfort yourself when you are tied up in your own obsessive, worrisome thoughts is to share them with another person whose support you know will be unstinting. Other people's responses can often comfort you, even at the simple level of interrupting the repetitious flow of your personal and habitual thought patterns. In the early days of my arthritis suffering, when my pain level was at its worst, I used to wake up in excruciating agony. My first trip down the hallway to the bathroom in the morning was an ordeal. I was in such pain, I moaned and complained the whole way, calling on God and my dead mother to comfort me and extend mercy. Sometimes I just moaned to express my anguish. Finally, my husband and young son protested to me. My husband said it was a horrible start to his day, to listen to my misery as I walked down the hall. My little boy said, "Mommy, I can't stand to hear you hurt so much, and I can't help you!" It broke my heart to hear him talk that way.

But I couldn't just give up my moaning and complaining. I felt they helped me bear the unbearable. To call out, to express my great distress. How could I endure such suffering in silence? I said to them, "I'm sorry, but I think I can't give it up. I will feel even worse. What will we do?"

My husband had a brilliant idea. He said, "Why don't we try answering you when you moan? That way, at least we'll be included rather than just listening to you and feeling helpless."

From then on, when I walked down the hall, groaning, crying out, I would hear sympathetic—and sometimes just communicative—whimpers, groans, and cries from my two guys. A long moan from me and then an answering lament from my husband with a lilt at the end, signifying a question, a request for information. Another deep wail from me, answering in the affirmative: yes, I hurt. A melodramatic drawn-out bawl from my son, wanting to be included. I gladly bellowed back to him, and so it continued down the hall, our entire household erupting in wails and shrieks. By the time I got to the bathroom, my heart was full. Such a container of sympathy and conversation for my travail. This never failed to make my heart sing, my eyes fill with gratitude and love. My two men reported how much they enjoyed moaning with me, how their helplessness had subsided. They cried out their own pain in being my witnesses as well as their sympathy for me.

Distraction: Down 'n' Dirty Comfort

Even though it's an ideal time to "embrace the suffering" or learn to "dance with disaster," you don't care. Furthermore, you don't care that you don't care. You've had it with trying to expand your consciousness. You hate your life and everybody in it. Nobody else cares; why should you? You're at the end of your rope. It's time for down 'n' dirty comfort. What you need is whatever will get you through the next few hours.

I think when things get this bad, you might have to start with a refuge, a place to which to retreat when you can't cope—just to find out what relief feels like. Once you know what relief feels like, you want to learn how to repeat it at will. When I first started to work on my healing, my therapist suggested that I look all over my body for a space that didn't hurt. When I protested that every part of me hurt, he insisted that I find a place without pain to which I could go when I needed to. I finally found it in my chest. Whenever I became overwhelmed with my pain or despair, I went to that spot in my chest and curled up into it as a cat lies down in the sun. So I started my healing process with a refuge, a port from the storm, a place to which to retreat when things got too hard. I think that if you can pay enough attention to locate your refuge, you can learn to locate your personal resources as well.

I think it's useful to search out and refine a place of refuge from your pain and stress, as I looked for a place to relax in my otherwise painful body. Think about what you use to comfort yourself when you are in unrelenting pain or overwhelmed by stress. You might consider making a list of these things to bring them further into your awareness. Don't hesitate to write down whatever it is, no matter how humiliating it might seem at first to think you actually need these silly things: mindless novels, trash TV, eating binges, complaining, punching a pillow, whatever. Of course, you can also include what are thought of as more wholesome modes of comfort, like petting your dog, writing poetry, inviting a friend to see a movie, and any comforting movements or stress-reduction exercises you may have learned.

When you list your sources of comfort this way, you develop an attitude similar to that with which you take down your prescription pain reliever from the shelf when you have a headache. You are aware that your pain or stress has become overwhelming, and you need to be comforted. Then when you curl up in an easy chair to read a romance novel, you have made a conscious decision to allow yourself to thoroughly enjoy the book. You can say to yourself, "I need comfort; I need to curl up, eat bonbons, and escape into a story that has nothing to do with my own troubles." That's very different from what people often do, which is guiltily read gossip magazines as a break from their real lives. It feels quite different to make a conscious decision to take time out from your everyday life and to do it wholeheartedly.

I have no trouble comforting myself any way I want since I have a degenerative, painful disease, and I work very hard. When I'm utterly miserable, beyond what a couple of ibuprofen will fix, I get into bed with a box of cookies and watch trash TV. I do it with complete consciousness and no guilt. Not, however, that I wouldn't be a little embarrassed if a friend actually caught me at it, *flagrante delicto*.

One particular Friday, I was exhausted, miserable, and resentful. I had worked hard all week, and it seemed to me that nobody appreciated me. Clients canceled their appointments, and nobody was taking any of my advice. My "poor me" tape started running, and my joints hurt. Although we were out of cookies, there were two Häagen-Dazs ice cream sandwiches in the fridge. I put them on a plate, curled up in bed under the thick comforter just the way I was, with my clothes and shoes on, and clicked on the TV. *Geraldo* was having a celebrity gossipfest with tabloid reporters telling all. I settled down into a blissful haze of pain, sugar, and gossip.

I was actually pretty transported, feeling much better about life, when the phone next to my bed rang a half hour later. Since I didn't want to go back into being-available mode, I had absolutely no intention of answering the phone or even listening to the message, but habit was stronger than gossip bliss. After the answering machine's various clicks indicated someone was beginning to record, I muted the TV at the last minute. A woman I didn't know began telling my machine she had heard me lecture and was very moved and impressed and wanted to study with me. I was such an inspiring person, she was sure forming a teaching relationship with me would help her cope with the pain she had in her life since I had set such an example with mine. She left her phone number. I clicked the TV mute button off and went back to *Geraldo*. In a few moments, I was laughing out loud. Here I was, the pain guru, the person people in pain want to emulate. I looked at myself huddled fully dressed under the bedcovers in the middle of the day, driven there by pain and self-pity, the plate full of ice cream sandwich crumbs sliding off to one side, my annoyance at having missed some Madonna gossip during the phone call, and thought, "*This is it.* This really *is* my teaching."

As Frank Sinatra reputedly said, "Whatever gets you through the night." I say if you're in real need, go for whatever gives your consciousness a little jiggle. But know what that is; know what your extremes are. Know what can debase you and what form your debasement takes. I think this is paradoxically very akin to fearlessness. It takes not a little courage to watch your whole process, the whole cycle. You go from being a high-functioning person dealing effectively with chronic pain to increasing irritability as you get more tired and the pain gets worse. Finally you're facing all-out defeat and inrushing despair. At this point, you choose comfort, even if that means depravity, and there's blessed spaciousness again before the pain starts anew. If you can watch this whole cycle—all without wincing, blinking, turning away, with your eyes open at every stage—you are a warrior.

PART TWO

DELIGHT

3

THE DISINTERESTED PURSUIT
OF PLEASURE

෴

W HEN we concern ourselves with the problem of chronic
pain, whether psychological or physical, we also need to
talk about pleasure. If we are in great pain, often the first step is
simply noticing that we have any pleasure at all in the midst of
terrible suffering. Then we need to learn how to notice that pleasure is actually present in the experience of pain. Not that pleasure distracts us from the pain or chases it away but that it is able
to send little tendrils of relief or comfort into the pain, in the
same way that darkness interpenetrates light, that death interpenetrates life.

I think that if you are overwhelmed by emotional stress or
physical pain, it is advisable to think about cultivating the ability
to recognize pleasure wherever the potential for its existence may
lie. I say this not because I am a thrill-seeking hedonist but because somebody has to say it. Not so many Zen lecturers or stress-
reduction teachers or arthritis doctors do, so I have to fill the
breach.

You might think, "Oh, she's wrong. Our culture places great
emphasis on pleasure. Just look at TV commercials, magazine
ads, our preoccupation with youth, and the general frivolity of
our society." The cultural values promoted by ad agencies are
not, however, quite what I mean by pleasure. We certainly are
encouraged to consume, but that is not exactly the same as being
encouraged to have pleasure. We are exhorted to purchase new

cars and to overextend ourselves buying gadgets on credit; we aren't really invited to baldly enjoy ourselves, to put our urge to sleep or dance or play ahead of our duties, or even to stretch or yawn or move our hips in public. It is against the law to take drugs, even privately, that merely increase our pleasure rather than relieve pain. So I do have to say something about pleasure, because I think doing something just for the plain old joy of doing it gets a bum rap in our culture.

This is especially true when enjoyment involves our bodies. We're still puritanical in many ways, and our bodies are considered dangerous. We demand the firing of a surgeon general because she doesn't condemn masturbation. The pope has warned Catholics against the practices of yoga and meditation specifically because they're body-based. The implication is that once we slip into the body, feel the sensual quality of its being, its urges, we may get swallowed up in that mode of perceiving forever. We might even fail to show up for work. I think we still have some remnant of that kind of prejudice, and physical pleasure is painted with the same brush of suspicion and disapproval as sensuality is. Also, many people who believe that a spiritual path includes suppression of the unpredictable urges of the corporeal self find they are so judgmental toward themselves that they immediately become locked in a battle against their own natures. It may be that what we need is to respect all the various aspects of our rich, multidimensional selves and learn the value of each of them, including our immensely serviceable inclination to have fun. So I'd like to propose that cultivating pleasure has a respectable and even necessary role in any spiritual practice.

It would be useful to first explore the relationship between pleasure and pain. Like a lot of pairs—light-dark, life-death, love-hate, sickness-health—pleasure and pain are interdependent. That is, they have meaning only in relation to each other. Our ability to perceive each of them is totally dependent on our understanding of the other. Their existence is so commingled in our consciousness that if we decide to concentrate our attention on one of them, the other comes into our consciousness eventually, whether we intend it or not. Sickness and health are an example I use often, because I work with people who have chronic physical problems.

When I began to recuperate from the worst ravages of rheumatoid arthritis, and spent more and more time out of my bed, I climbed onto the ever-turning wheel of the sickness-health dichotomy. Every morning when I awoke, I'd think, "Am I better or worse today?" Because I was emotionally involved with the answer—I was repelled by my sickness and clinging to any signs of good health—I was either cast down and disappointed, or raised up and elated, depending on whether I was feeling better or worse.

You don't have to be particularly ill to get caught up in this cycle. You can just decide to improve your health by dieting or exercising or going on a special program. You work very hard at improving yourself. You take vitamins and watch your diet and work out. You get on the scale and compare your weight to the day before, or you see whether you can run farther than you did last week, and so on. Things go well for a time, and you feel better, your clothes fit better, you have more stamina.

But then you start to notice when you don't feel so good. You overtrained yesterday, so now you have some minor aches and pains. You went to a party one night and picked up a pound or two on the scale the next morning. It starts to drive you crazy that one little deviation from your regimen can make such a difference. It becomes worrisome because now you're not only noticing when you feel very good, you're also noticing more than you ever did before when you don't feel absolutely tip-top. When you plucked "feeling good" out of the undiscriminated void—that is, when you decided to direct your attention to feeling good—you didn't realize that you were going to start noticing "feeling worse" as well. Whenever you become preoccupied with relative states, you're vulnerable to the sudden manifestation of one of them or the other. You're cast down or raised up—you experience pain or pleasure—with very little provocation: the reading on a scale, the fit of a pair of pants, or the ability to move your leg a little more or less than you did yesterday. It's not the original decision to change something about yourself that becomes the problem; it's your attachment to the outcome.

So the significant difference between pleasure and pain is the emotion each of them elicits. We're usually repelled by pain and attracted to pleasure. If we observe the circularity of these feelings often enough, however—how disappointment and elation follow each other over and over—we begin to see their essential unity. They have the same source, the same root in the human psyche: our primeval tendency to grasp pleasure and avoid pain. Neither of them can stand alone; they only have meaning in relation to each other. It's the emotion we put on each of them that makes them stand out in our lives.

The relationship between pleasure and pain can get very muddy. We can have an attraction or an aversion to both pleasure and pain. Either pleasure or pain can change into the other, often without our even noticing the precise moment when that happens. For example, when we talk to others about our suffering, we often feel relieved. Joy floods in to such an extent that we're embarrassed by suddenly feeling very light in the middle of describing our great suffering. We actually seem to get pleasure from acknowledging our pain. Where does suffering end and delight start?

We have all had the experience of going to a celebration and seeing with great pleasure the tables groaning with delicious things to eat and drink. We dive into the feast, giving ourselves permission to eat everything we want on this special day. We eat and eat, and it's all wonderful; it's great. The champagne makes us lighthearted and vivacious. But in a very short time, we have this terrible heavy, bloated feeling that prevents us from dancing or enjoying the rest of the party. The champagne makes our heads throb, and we feel really bad. At which forkful did pleasure turn into pain? At which sip from our glass?

It's the same thing with love and hate, another pair that turn into each other with alarming and unpredictable frequency. Many women comment that they have come to hate the very trait that attracted them to a new boyfriend in the first place. In the beginning, he seemed so quiet and sensitive, not loud and macho like other men. But a few months later, "quiet and sensitive" has turned into "never shares his feelings." Similarly, the friend who is fun because she is constantly effervescent and upbeat becomes exhausting after a few hours.

It's not their fault; these people didn't change after you met them. The problem lies in your focus on and response to a particular personality trait. Out of all this person's ten thousand characteristics, you singled out one to be hung up on. What you now find so irritating is just the underbelly of what attracted you to begin with. You started the cycle of clinging-aversion when you chose to focus on a particular character trait and make it more important than any other. You held fast to the positive aspect of that characteristic and imbued it with enormous value, your estimation of your lover or friend. "Quiet" is positive, desirable. But once you focus so intently on one trait, you are vulnerable to perceiving the other pole, "remote," because opposites depend on each other for meaning. The preoccupation with one side of the pair has turned on you. So the problem with pain is aversion, and the problem with pleasure is clinging.

The solution is to just live your life without getting tripped up by all these fixations, but "just" means living your whole life. It's being alive for all the details of your life and not picking out the moments that you're going to attend to and those you're going to ignore. You can take care of your body simply because it yearns to be taken care of and you are alive, listening to its yearnings, flowing in and out of its intelligence, not making it into a separate being apart from yourself. You can attend to your relationships with friends and mates with a heart open to all their various characteristics, those you enjoy and those you find annoying. There is an absence of struggle when you pay attention this way. What is really going on is that you are doing what needs to be done for your body and for your relationships; it's not you against sickness or pain or your friends' personalities.

When you do prefer one state of mind over another, whether it's pleasure or pain, you lose your capacity to be present in the moment. When you're making love, you're taking time out to think, "Can we do this again before morning?" Instead of tasting every morsel in your mouth during the birthday dinner lovingly prepared by your friends, you're thinking, "What's the next course?" You're constantly living somewhere else, in the past or the future.

If you do see your cycle of craving and aversion, and regard it with some humor or detachment, bemused at the fact that you're always running after something or away from something, you can begin to practice the *disinterested* pursuit of pleasure. This is pleasure recognized and fostered rather than frantically and compulsively grasped at. You can cultivate pleasure in the same way that you eat sensibly or put on your jacket when it's cold. This is just something you do for your and others' well-being.

Why should you cultivate pleasure in this disinterested way? Recent research indicates that pleasure is good for you. Pleasure is biochemically better for your health than pain is; it produces a different blood chemistry than pain does. Pleasurable experiences make you breathe deeper, and some of them make your immune system function better. Pleasure relaxes your body, so that your muscles are more flexible and responsive. They can gently pull your joints apart as you move, keeping you from getting arthritis or easing the arthritis you already have.

Having pleasure can also make you kind and generous toward yourself and others, which is important for your long-term satisfaction and happiness. If you feel that your life is bountiful, that your needs are met, then you naturally feel like sharing the overflow. That's true generosity, not social convention.

I know firsthand about the difference between real generosity and social convention because I came to Zen practice thinking I was a generous person. I always gave to people on the street, and whenever anybody asked me to help do something, I gave him or her my best effort. But after staying at the San Francisco Zen Center for some time, I discovered that my generosity was pretty shallow. At Zen Center, the demands for assistance in the kitchen, in the office, and in cleaning the large, beautiful building were so constant that I found myself hiding out, pretending to be unavailable, and resenting the fact that I seemed to be spending all my time helping other people rather than pleasing myself.

After a while, the gap between my social behavior and my real behavior got so large, it troubled me. I told my problem to a teacher at Zen Center, and he encouraged me to begin a selfishness practice to see where my true generosity might lie. So for the next several months, whenever cookies were served at tea, I was always very careful to take the largest one. Whenever anyone asked me for help with something, I always said no. This was very hard at first, but eventually I got into it. After some months, I felt so personally nourished that I found myself spontaneously offering to help someone almost without realizing it. I thought about it later and realized that I finally felt completely taken care of, that I was full to the brim, and so I was willing—even eager—to share my bounty with others. This is the internal revolution that turns the social convention of courteous helpfulness into genuine and unstinting generosity. In the realm of helping or nurturing behavior, charity very much begins at home.

Robert Aitken has described the perfection of charity as the realization that life is a wallet stuffed with hundred-dollar bills, but you have no thought of putting them into your pocket. I think you begin to cultivate this open and generous state of mind when you no longer feel compelled to stockpile the hundred-dollar bills. You can grin at your own impulse to gather the bills, the joys of life, and hold them close against some future misery or to impulsively spend them for fear this will be your only chance to experience such plenitude. When you have become perceptive enough to recognize your own pleasure in every event and encounter, in every difficulty and challenge, you know better. You can feel your whole life strewn with hundred-dollar bills, with satisfaction and abundance. When you have this much faith in your ability to perceive and nurture your own joy, you also begin to feel generous toward your own tendency to be caught in the cycle of grasping and aversion. If you are able to extend your charity to the aspects of yourself you know cause you pain, you are developing the broad and generous spirit of letting everything be what it is, including yourself.

ASPECTS OF PLEASURE

As a person with a chronic illness who works with other people who have long-term physical difficulties, I'm very interested in what we do that has some influence on our healing process. Over the years, I've noticed that among the most important healing experiences we can have are experiences of deep pleasure. When our suffering is chronic or intense, we cannot let our pleasures come randomly. We need to take the perception of pleasure very seriously and learn how to build the occurrence of such feelings into our lives.

What are the experiences that are so pleasurable that they transform us? In the following chapters, I will discuss various aspects of pleasure that I have come to regard as crucial for the biochemical and psychological alleviation of suffering:

- Engagement with life, a feeling of being in charge (Chapter 4)
- Ecstasy as refreshment (Chapter 5)
- Nurturing relationships (Chapter 6)
- Relaxation and movement (Chapter 8)

Incorporating movement and relaxation, pleasant body feelings, and even ecstasy, the temporary suspension of the boundaries of time and space, into your daily life is deeply healing for your body and indescribably refreshing to your mind. All have profound potential for giving you the perspective to free yourself from everyday stresses and chronic pain. Once you have altered the way you spend your days to include some of these practices, you may be brought low by your life circumstances, but you'll never again be trapped in just the same way. What this kind of attention introduces is spaciousness, space around thoughts and activities that allows you to live a rich and satisfying life right in the middle of misery.

4

CONTROLLING YOUR SHEEP OR COW IN THE LARGE, SPACIOUS MEADOW

～

Long ago a monk asked the old master, "When hundreds, thousands or myriads of objects come all at once, what should be done?"
The master replied, "Don't try to control them."
—ZEN MASTER DOGEN

PAIN AND SUFFERING
THE ISSUE OF CONTROL

WE devote our lives to attempts to avoid pain and create pleasure. Sometimes we even appear to be successful. We may avoid adversity for a long time, only to discover that when something terrible breaks through our carefully maintained protective strategies, the pain is all the more intense for our being unaccustomed to its pangs. I have noticed that if I go for some time without a disaster—that is, nothing particularly disappointing occurs for some days or weeks—then when something does happen to shake me out of my pleasant routine, I am undone. It's as if I've forgotten the rhythms of suffering. I've fallen asleep. As unwilling as I am at first to wake up and face the calamity, when I finally do so, I always feel invigorated, as if someone had just splashed a huge pan of cold salt water over me.

Have you ever spent time in a room full of people who, for one reason or another, have not suffered grossly for a very long time? People who might have the financial resources to avoid even witnessing really terrible suffering like lying drunk on the sidewalk or being without a secure place to sleep or having enough food or fearing the predators who wait for you to fall asleep at night? Some people have been able to limit their discomfort to much more subtle varieties, like not being able to get something they would like to have, for a long time. Not that their suffering is different in degree, but it mostly takes place in very refined realms, such as aesthetic disappointments or temporary personal hindrances. They may get very upset over an irritating neighbor who builds a structure that blocks their view or get emotionally involved in rescuing their plants from garden pests. There's not much vitality in a room full of such people; the feeling of enervation is palpable. When I'm in a situation like this, I always feel like putting on rap music full volume or something, just to get some juice flowing.

People who live in comfortable circumstances need not be distanced from gross forms of suffering—many such people are horrified by others' circumstances and work hard to help—but those who can isolate themselves often choose to do so. And sometimes the price of this isolation is disconnection, a gradual loss of a broad perspective from which to regard our own and others' human pain. For this reason, my husband and I prefer to live in a city, although we love the countryside with its peace and beauty. The city is ground zero for suffering. If homeless and sick people and mistreated children are going to do some kind of extreme suffering, I want it to be under my nose. I don't want to be disconnected from it.

On the other hand, we don't have to be rich to tightly control our awareness of our own and others' suffering. We can avoid newspapers, TV, and any other kind of communication that threatens to blast us with unnecessary unpleasantness. Even if we can't afford to live in a gated community, we can isolate ourselves from any possible disruption of our state of mind; we can admit only the most reserved and well-behaved persons into our company. We can routinize our lives so thoroughly that little is left to chance. In other words, we may be able to exert a great deal of control by making our world very small. I think some amount of containment is necessary to live a life that is ordered enough to allow us to function well, to enjoy our maximum energy, to have sufficient peace of mind to treat each other respectfully. But many of us go too far, organizing our lives to such an extent that nothing threatening, or even spontaneous and refreshing, could ever happen to us. Our world gets narrower and narrower until we start to feel lifeless, isolated from others.

It seems to me that one of life's most challenging aspects for all of us is how to limit the amount of stress and pain we experience without giving up the possibility of adventure. Restricting the amount of misery we're personally aware of, as described above, is one strategy. But we have to be careful here. There is a huge price tag if we go too far: we lose touch with some of life's most vital experiences—those of fear, uncertainty, of spontaneous contact with strangers. How do we minimize our suffering without excessive controlling, without shutting down our lives completely by strangling the vitality out of them with our need to control the flow of events? And on the other hand, how do we know when to seize the day—to go for it, to take risks that bring us real and important pleasures: a sense of empowerment, ecstasy, relationship? Where is it we must make an effort to bring things under control, and where is it we should let go and just allow? How can we learn to tell the difference?

Some of us are naturally controlling types. We can't notice or observe anything without interfering with it somehow. When I asked students in a stress-reduction class to put their attention on their breathing, one woman found herself unable to focus on her breath and breathe naturally at the same time. When she paid close attention to her breathing, mindful of her inhalations and exhalations, she interfered with its natural rhythm. She tended to take over the inhalations and exhalations with her conscious mind, making them longer, and then panicking because she felt as if she wasn't getting enough air. Finally, she resorted to counting her heartbeats—so many to inhale, so many to exhale—in order to allow her breathing to continue in a regular fashion. This woman had the ability to focus her mind and the determination to sit herself down to meditate regularly, but once seated, she couldn't stop controlling herself. She needed to learn how and when to get out of the way and just allow her breath to come and go on its own. Focusing on her problem in this very specific way not only helped her to get out of the way of her breath but enabled her to discover how to "get out of the way" in other realms of her life as well. The observations she made of her own behavior in our stress-reduction class transformed her ability to, as she put it, "take care of what needs to be taken care of, allow what needs to arise by itself, and know the difference!"

The feeling of having some kind of control in our lives is very important to our health and well-being. In *Healing and the Mind,* Dean Ornish talks about the biochemical importance of empowerment, the fact that taking responsibility for our own health and well-being, as opposed to handing ourselves over passively to a medical professional, has a positive effect on the biochemistry of our body's systems. So it seems very important for us to believe that we are basically in charge, to feel that we can act and produce results by acting. Perhaps one of the most important aspects of pleasure in its broadest meaning is our sense that we have some sort of control—*mastery* might be a better word—over our lives.

The extent to which we can exercise control over the amount of discomfort in our lives has a profound effect on physical as well as mental health. Scientists believe the factor responsible for the built-in stress in some jobs is a feeling of loss of control. When workers are given wide responsibilities combined with a lack of personal control over how work is done, their health is adversely affected. People who develop a degenerative disease also experience loss of control with respect to their health and the functioning of their bodies. Their first realization is that they can no longer order their bodies around as they once could. In the arthritis workshops I have led, people talk most about their loss of control, the betrayal of their bodies. This seems to be a major issue for people with serious illness.

It would appear that deciding to take the major responsibility for our own healing and to seek the advice and treatment of medical professionals as consultants is crucial if we have a long-term chronic illness. From my experience with my own body and from observing people I teach, I have come to believe that there is some biochemical concomitant of active, conscious, deliberate attempts to heal ourselves, beginning with relaxation techniques that seem to enable us to pick up the body's signals through the garble of goal-oriented thoughts and panic over our condition. This is not to say I oppose consultation with and treatment from physicians. I just think it is probably not conducive to our health and psychological well-being to become passively dependent on health-care providers or drugs.

When we feel in control of our physical well-being and our pain level, as a result of eventually coming to know our body and our affliction intimately, even a flare-up of our condition will have less impact on us than on someone who is dependent on another person for his or her ease. We know that we ourselves can work through any setback or recover any temporarily lost function. A person in a helpless stance, by contrast, will be overwhelmed by fear and panic, further aggravating an already toxic situation.

JUST THE RIGHT AMOUNT OF CONTROL

So, then, what is just the right touch, the right orchestration of our circumstances without too much control or too much looseness? What is the right kind and right amount of effort to make? When do you make an effort to affect situations, and when do you step back and let things flow as they will?

Many of us tend to bombard a difficult situation with compulsive and blind effort that buries its particulars in all the flailing about. Making much too much effort all the time in every situation is not only exhausting, but it is a way of avoiding true engagement with our lives. We're so involved in our response, we can't tell what's actually going on in the situation we're reacting to. This strategy has all the earmarks of panic. We strive and we struggle and we apply ourselves utterly, which eliminates all opportunities to actually experience the often distressing hills and gullies of a demanding situation.

My own experience of doing this is that it protects me from feeling my fear at not being able to handle the situation; I can't bear to actually feel that twinge of terror that seizes my stomach, especially if the outcome of my effort is important. It makes me feel more in control if my focus is unswervingly on the feeling of struggle itself, not on the details of living through it or the end result. When I get into this mode, I feel as if I'm fighting my way through a blizzard, struggling against the cold, strong wind that is freezing me as I'm trying to reach my destination, my cozy little cabin with a fire going inside where I can finally rest. So I fight and struggle, gasping as the wind takes my breath away, bravely planting each foot in the deep snow, my head down against the roaring wind, and eventually I realize I passed my warm little cabin a long time ago. I've thrown myself into the effort and have forgotten why.

Revving yourself up to tackle a difficult project you really don't want to do at all is like this. After you summon the energy required, your ongoing effort is directed toward keeping the energy up. You don't check in on the big picture, the context of the project, and see what it needs, stage by stage, maybe because that would require coming out of a static emotional stance and tuning in to your feelings enough to evaluate the situation and make value judgments at very specific and particular times. If you just rev up and blitz through the situation without pausing for judgment or feeling, you miss all its hills and gullies, its subtleties. Even though it's hard to maintain this kind of tension for any length of time, many people find it easier than experiencing what may be for them a deep, visceral distaste for their activity.

A friend of mine did this for some months in order to handle a difficult labor situation at the company where she is vice president. Two months later, after the conflict had been resolved by a professional mediator, she was physically drained and spiritually demoralized. She realized she had put herself in an emotionally neutral holding pattern so that she could go through that situation without noticing how angry it made her. She was chagrined to realize she could actually have handled it much more deftly, with less cost to herself, if she had been more aware and accepting of how the situation had made her feel. She had behaved throughout as if it were just one kind of event, labor against management, instead of becoming attuned to its subtleties, the individuals involved, and their different agendas.

Anyone looking at her would never have guessed that every part of her being was not wholly engaged; she was right in the middle of things, rendering decisions and barking orders. But administrators and staff alike found it impossible to relate to her. She was not accessible emotionally. Her lack of emotional engagement, and the true fury behind it, was covered up by indiscriminant effort. She was flailing madly rather than negotiating effectively. She was making too much of the wrong kind of effort, compulsive and headlong, burying the details of the situation in frenetic activity.

Others of us are undone before we start; we sweep difficult situations under the rug and ignore the bulge. This is another way to avoid real engagement in our lives. If we feel instantly overwhelmed in a situation, we're usually viewing it in its total aggregate: its complexity, its threat to us. If we never settle down enough to pick out any details to engage with, we won't find any access point into mastery of the situation. We're blitzed; we protect ourselves by just giving up immediately. Of course, we don't put it to ourselves that way exactly. We'll say to ourselves and our friends that the situation is not worthy of our time, or we're too busy doing something important, or we don't want to get involved with those kinds of people. This stance takes a different kind of emotional toll from revving up: we feel enervation, a lack of vitality, a sense that we just don't have enough energy to effectively meet the problems of our complex lives. And over time, we begin to resent this kind of stress, imposed on us as it is from the intruding outside world, so that more and more of our vital energy is tied up in the feelings of events being beyond our control.

I remember a time when I was afraid to go through the mail every day because it often contained demands to cope with complex situations that I saw as blatantly personal attacks on me by the universe: a credit card balance that included an annual fee the company had assured me it wouldn't charge; a telephone bill with calls I hadn't made or services I hadn't ordered; a notice from the state of California that it is revising the tax laws concerning sales of audiotapes (which I sell); junk mail announcing that my car insurance costs much more than it needs to—and its claims sounded worthy of interrupting my life and investigating; an envelope from the Department of Motor Vehicles addressed to my son (who often borrows my car); a threat to sue me for payment of a medical bill I thought I had paid ages ago—so long ago, I no longer had the canceled check.

Our modern lives are very complicated. Just maintaining a household as simple as mine involves a variety of corporations, government agencies, and service industries, all with vast potential to make obstinate and persistent errors in their accounting, as well as various arbitrary demands on me, solely because I have a mailbox. The stack of mail on the hall table at the end of the week was staggering until I made it a practice to sit down with a cup of tea and go through it several times a week, sorting it into piles to be tossed, handled immediately, or handled whenever I feel like it. The "handled immediately" items get tacked onto the list of phone calls I make each morning and will probably be addressed in the next few days. The "handled whenever I feel like it" items, such as inquiries into new services, will eventually be seen to as my leisure and interest level permit. In other words, I have transformed that previously unassailable stack of demands, errors, and calculated evil into a relaxing teatime (which I always felt I didn't get often enough) during which I alternately curse the invention of the printing press and chuckle with delight (we do also occasionally get mail that we welcome—from friends who are vacationing or making invitations or announcing accomplishments).

We often experience this kind of overwhelm and frustration with the complex and legalistic situations that arise in today's world. When I went to Seattle to visit a longtime buddy who has moved there from California, she was in the middle of an energy-sapping dilemma about her car. Another car had hit hers and wrecked it. She couldn't drive it. Although, at the scene, the other driver had admitted being in the wrong, she later contradicted herself to her insurance adjuster. Thus, the other driver's insurance company refused to pay. My friend felt completely undone by the other driver's dishonesty as well as overwhelmed by the idea that someone could just by chance alter her life so profoundly.

In a very tired and dejected little voice, she told me that she just wanted to get on with her life, to start brainstorming ideas to raise money to replace her car. When I suggested calling a lawyer and finding out whether she had a case, she resisted, saying she didn't want to get even more involved with unscrupulous people. Look what she had already had to deal with. But I pressed her until she did agree to call a lawyer recommended by a friend.

Fortunately, the lawyer provided the access point that she needed to enter the situation she had found so overwhelming. He explained to her that if she decided to retain him, there were several junctures at which she could discontinue the case: if she thought it was costing too much, it was unethical, or even just that she was losing. As she considered the possibility of taking this situation on, she realized that diving into it meant that she was going to fully feel her outrage at having been victimized and perhaps even being cheated in the end. As we talked, she indeed began to express her anger; I felt her energy level rise. But she saw the creative possibilities. By the time she called the lawyer with her decision to proceed, she was engaged and assertive.

She said to me later on the phone after our visit that the main thing that intrigued her about this suit was the idea that seeing it through required her to be awake and alert to its nuances whenever it changed. If she simply let the lawyer handle it all, she would feel uneasy, but with just the right amount of attentive persistence, she could make some good decisions and feel as if she was participating in her own fate, no matter what the outcome. She said she was going to reinforce this practice of appreciating each step of the way with the practice of not reaching for toilet paper until the flow of her pee stopped. "Do you get it?"

she asked me. Of course, she meant she was taking it one step at a time, doing one thing after another, being completely engaged in each activity until it ended and the next one began.

A woman I know who owns her own successful business began a meditation practice after a family crisis led her to believe she was unaware of much of her motivation in interpersonal matters. She found meditation practice extremely relaxing, since she was able to put aside her everyday cares and focus her mind on her breath and body. After just a few months of such practice, she realized that she rarely relaxed outside of her regular meditation period. Although she claimed to love her daily work of creating shoe designs that would later be manufactured and supervising her employees, she admitted that every work morning it was necessary to rev herself up to go to work. There was nothing "natural" about her effort. She couldn't go from a leisurely morning cup of tea to arriving at her desk ready to work. She needed first to put herself in "work mode," a state of heightened urgency and nervous energy, before flinging herself at her tasks. Then, at the end of the day, she collapsed, barely able to interact with her children at dinner let alone pursue the nightlife she had intended to enjoy after her divorce.

When she tried to take her meditation state of mind into her workplace, it evaporated at the first glimpse of her desk. She was impressed with how persistent her habit of urgent overkill was, even when she wanted to break it. Finally she decided to treat the issue of her effort like a koan, a question that she asked herself over and over again in all kinds of situations: "What is the right effort in this situation? What is the right amount of attention and energy that I need to bring to this situation in order to do what needs to be done here, step after step? How can I do just that without adding anything extra to the real effort I need to make?"

A few weeks into asking herself that question periodically during her day, she was in despair. The plug had been pulled. Without the feeling that she was always staving off imminent disaster, she felt no drive to do her work. She realized that her usual high drive level made her feel powerful and able to meet the complex demands of her business. Without it, she feared she would never do anything again. She said to me, genuinely frightened, "I guess I don't have any basic motivation to do anything at all." But when I saw her a week later, she was starting to feel her own real engine beginning to chug. Freed of the habit of being driven by her fantasies of ultimate ruin, she was able to feel her own natural energy and inclination. She had gotten in touch with the yearnings of her own creativity.

To foster the feeling that you have things under control, it may be necessary to allow the elements of the universe you previously thought of as being beyond your control to come onto the racetrack with you as your partners rather than your chattel. Let loose of the reins a little bit so that you and your horses can participate together in establishing your realm of control. Let your teenager help decide his or her own curfew. Include your employees or coworkers in decisions about the company or your job that may affect them. Let your mate have activities or friends that don't interest or include you. This is a more porous conception of control than we are used to.

Shunryu Suzuki, founder of the San Francisco Zen Center, remarks in *Zen Mind, Beginner's Mind:*

> To give your sheep or cow a large, spacious meadow is the way to control him. It's the same with taking care of your everyday life. Even though you try to put people under some control, it is impossible. . . . Just . . . watch them without trying to control them. . . . It is the same with various images you have in your mind. Let them come and let them go. Then they will be under control. . . . The true purpose of zen is to see things as they are and to let everything go as it goes. This is to put everything under control in its widest sense.

A big part of what you must learn if you're to be less worried about controlling everything is how to let go of your compulsive need to feel in control. You would be better off making the effort it takes to learn when to stop making effort, when to allow things to just happen, to simply let your impulses come forth. This is the art of cultivating faith in your intuition, learning to trust in your inherent wisdom.

NOT-KNOWING MIND

Because, of course, in reality, you don't have control over your life. You may be clever enough to set up situations to maximize your pleasure, or you may take actions that cause events to occur, but you can't cover all the bases. Human life is just too vast, way beyond your imagination. You can try your best: you can wear your seat belts to protect yourself in case of an auto accident or put up a gate so your child doesn't fall down the stairs, but you may not be able to avoid that accident, and your child may get hurt some other way. You can't control the circumstances of your birth, the way you grow up, most other people's behavior, the course your life will take, or the timeless procession of human sorrow.

If you live or work with other people, you soon realize how emotionally unpredictable human beings are. People are launched into the emotional stratosphere by seemingly trivial re-marks or events. You're likely to notice especially that other peo-ple are this way, though you can't predict your own reactions 100 percent either. If you doubt my words, observe your thoughts for a few minutes while trying to focus your mind on one thing—say, your breath. You will start to get a feel for how little control you actually have over your own mind. If you are not accustomed to noticing the jumble of thoughts that occupy your waking mind, you will probably be amazed that you can ever gather a few simi-lar ones together for long enough to carry out the simplest task. The first thing you're struck with when you begin to watch your thoughts is how unmanageable they are. They scoot from thing to thing like a curious puppy let off a leash.

If you begin to notice the particulars of your own thought process, you discover how repetitious and habit-based its individ-ual patterns are, how hard it is for you to experiment with the focus of your usual thinking and deviate the least little bit from the patterns to which your mind is already accustomed. For instance, you might start to do some stress-reduction practices, such as learning to breathe deeply at certain times during the day with your full attention on your breath rather than on your computer screen. Practices like this are very difficult to establish because they go against the usual flow of your thoughts. It's like sticking a frail pole in a rushing river. You understand from these attempts at interrupting your usual flow patterns how little mastery you actually have over your own mind, let alone the rest of the universe. If you can't control the workings of your own mind, how can you expect to influence anything outside of yourself, let alone how much pain and pleasure you have in your life?

In Zen, this is called "not-knowing" mind. Dainin Katagiri, a modern-day Zen master who taught many years at the Minneapolis Zen Center, said:

> As long as you are a human being, you are right in the middle of the situation of not understanding anything because life is vast, because it is the truth. Truth or vastness or emptiness is very rich but you cannot name it. All you can do is to practice, receive and accept that full richness. There's no way to know this, but you are already there, so first accept this fact. The point you have to know is that you are right in the situation of not understanding anything.

My friend Daya calls this kindergarten mind: we're always at the beginning. With this attitude, we never get very stale or stray too far from our deep needs. We won't be one of the unfortunate people who reach old age before they suddenly awake from their numbness and cry, "What have I been doing? I've wasted my life!" Or even worse, who die without ever waking up to their real life, the life that awaited them beyond the expectations of others. Unfortunately, we humans are pretty uncomfortable with not knowing. We're always trying to extend our areas of expertise, to turn new situations into the old ones with which we're familiar and in which we have already excelled. Daya told me that her son Kelly was very anxious before starting school each year.

He would say, "Mom, I don't know how to do second grade."
Daya had to tell him, "You don't have to know how to do second
grade before you do second grade."

We always seem to need to be prepared because we are so
fearful of what's ahead. But knowing is comparatively static; not
knowing is the creative space. Not knowing allows an opening, a
new event, some notion rising from our own unconscious, some
original face. This is learning to respect and enjoy the inherent
wisdom we've cultivated in our disciplined spiritual practice or
we've noticed has developed during our examined life. I believe
that developing the capacity to tolerate not-knowing mind allows
what we call "intuition" to evolve. This is the metabolite of body
wisdom, the availability to our conscious minds of the benefits of
the insight and experience assimilated by both body and mind in
all our years of making choices and allowing opportunities.

This was brought home dramatically for me several years ago,
after I had been living and working at the San Francisco Zen
Center for about fifteen years. I arranged to spend some time at
Tassajara, Zen Center's mountain monastery in glorious Big Sur,
during the summer, when the monastery opens its hot springs
and rustic cabins to guests. My daily job at Zen Center involved a
great deal of administrative responsibility, so it was a very nice
break to go to Tassajara and just clean cabins for incoming guests
in the morning, swim and sun in the afternoon, and sit meditation at night.

After I had been at Tassajara for about ten days, some kind
of turmoil started in my mind. Not actual thoughts, but strange
feelings and images. I had the sense, regardless of where I actually was, of being in a close, dark, warm space, almost like a birth
canal. After a few more days in which these images intensified,
my inner world became more compelling than my outer world. I
was attuned to it no matter what I was doing, even conversing
with another person. I also felt uncharacteristically passive. I was
in the receive mode for these images and feelings. I felt no urge
to act on them or even to struggle to make sense of them. As the
days went by, these feelings became so imposing that they caused
me to withdraw from social activities at Tassajara; my interactions

just didn't seem as real as my feelings. I started eating alone and being alone in my cabin whenever I wasn't working. This was very unusual behavior for me, and eventually I became afraid, wondering what was happening to me.

Even though I was afraid, I didn't think I was going insane. Years of meditation enabled me to trust the workings of my own mind, even if they were unfamiliar. I sensed that something was coming up to my consciousness from below, something that had found an opportunity, while my focus was relatively loose and relaxed at Tassajara, to get my attention.

That experience was the first stage of a big change in my life that initially stirred inside me and then worked its way up into my consciousness and out into the world. The feelings that came up continued to be so strong that I wholly gave myself over to them and let them direct my life. I had the sense of channeling powerful impulses rather than of making up my mind what to do. Soon after I returned to the city, I decided without understanding why that I should leave my monastic life at Zen Center and reenter the world of jobs and material concerns. In retrospect, it seems that after so many years of self-examination in Zen Center, I needed to shift into a more active mode, from gathering in to bursting out, from the contemplative to the ecstatic. At the time, though, I could only follow my intuition. The strange yearnings and images at Tassajara were a great opening for me, a broadening of my understanding of what is the right effort to make, the art of knowing when to act and when to allow. I was quite struck by the necessity of allowing, following, receiving, and trusting in that.

I think we Americans are particularly uncomfortable with that not-knowing realm. We're problem solvers; we're doers; in our country's young history, we've never taken no for an answer. A mere 150 years ago, early Americans were conquering an indigenous people and developing a vast continent of raw resources into an economy to support huge numbers of immigrant peoples. Every generation since the turn of the century has grown up in considerably different material and cultural circumstances than the one before it. What could we not control or conquer?

In the stress-reduction classes I conduct at hospitals, people sometimes protest that I'm not giving them a series of solid, easily grasped techniques to reduce stress. Instead, it's just this nebulous meditation practice. Some people are extremely uncomfortable with this and wonder whether they're learning anything useful. It's very hard for most of us to think about anything without being goal-directed. We see our stress as a problem to be overcome and eliminated, like hemorrhoids. We want to reduce stress, plain and simple, not merge with it, not study it, not hold it in meditative equipoise. We think that whatever we're going to learn to conquer our stress, it should be definite, graspable. It's difficult for us to live in the realm of not knowing, just giving everything in front of us our whole attention and suspending our worry about what comes next until it arrives. We need to cultivate a lot of faith to live that way. But this attitude may be the most intimate and satisfying connection we could ever have with our lives. Not to know exactly what's going to happen but to do, to feel, anyway.

As for me, I find that the not-knowing space is definitely part of my creative process. When I'm working on a particular problem I'm trying to solve, whether it be how to schedule the activities in a workshop or how to comfort a client in pain, the experimental attitude, the not-knowing mind, the tentative mind that will entertain many possibilities, is very satisfying space for me. Yes, I love the illusion of certainty, that solid, no-nonsense, take-charge feeling. But what a breather when my thoughts rummage freely in my mind, loosened for a time from their usually tight mooring to their little tried-and-true categories. If we can learn to be at all comfortable with that state of mind, we certainly will come to value its true and accurate relationship to the realities of this life.

RAISING THE BANNER OF TRUTH

Maybe the closest we get to control or mastery is in the sense that Dean Ornish meant, that we can engage ourselves, meet our lives right where we are, whatever kind of life we currently have. What I'm talking about here is a much more subtle feeling than what we usually think of as control of our lives, in the sense that we can monitor or moderate what happens to us in some way. That's a little heavier-handed than I mean. I'm trying to convey the feeling we have when we feel totally involved in our lives; we feel completely used up, as if there were no separation between us and what we're doing. We may not be able to perfectly control what happens in our lives, but we can make an effort to be present for anything that does happen. We can penetrate our natural aversion toward our difficulties. We can cultivate our willingness to meet challenges and expand the energy level we have available to take them on. It costs us something to turn away from situations that come up. We become afraid, our energy level plummets, and we feel defeated. We do seem to need to feel that we can affect our lives in some intimate way and that the events and people in our lives can vibrate back, engaging us more and more until we can no longer meaningfully distinguish between ourselves and our ideas of what our lives should be. There is only the experience of activity.

Dainin Katagiri-roshi said that his teacher, Hashimoto-roshi, told him, "In whatever situation you may be in, in whatever place you are standing right here and now, this is the place in which you have to erect the banner of truth." Katagiri-roshi added, "This means the naked reality of being is full of richness, but you can't name it, you can't understand it. Your whole existence is completely embraced by this full richness, just like a baby held in its mother's arms. This is the naked reality of all beings."

What does he mean, to raise your own banner of truth wherever you are? I think this means to engage with your life, to embrace it wholeheartedly as it unfolds. Thus, it will always unfold according to your own nature.

My husband, Tony, decided to go to graduate school at about the same time I left to explore the world outside the monastery. Because we had been living and working at Zen Center in its various locations for nearly fifteen years, we were very disoriented by our new outside jobs and the constant company of people who had never practiced meditation. My husband worked as a real estate appraiser to pay his graduate school tuition, and I began using the massage and movement training I had learned to treat my own rheumatoid arthritis to offer treatment to paying clients. This was a very difficult transition for both of us. Because I was just reentering the world of business, my new clients very generously and kindly gave me lots of advice.

One told me I should dye my graying hair so I would look younger and therefore healthier because my profession involved health. I figured since she was in the business world, she knew what was best. So I followed her advice and dyed my hair back to its former dark brown. Another said I would eventually need a face-lift because the standards for appearance in the San Francisco Bay Area are so high. I was a little more dubious about that one. I thought, well, maybe I'll move to Oregon when my face gets too saggy. Another asked me whether I had established a college fund for our son. After all, she pointed out, that was only eight years away. We hadn't given a thought to any such thing. Another client asked me whether we had an IRA, adding that if you waited until your forties to start one, it would be too late to accumulate enough money for your retirement. (I was forty-two and my husband forty-four.) Another client said that if we didn't buy property right away (this was during the real estate boom of the eighties), we would be priced out of the Bay Area in ten years and not even be able to rent a place.

All this advice was very upsetting and confusing, and my husband and I began feeling frantic about our lives and how far behind we were in acquiring security and providing for our child. It upset me very much to think our chosen lifestyle might have shortchanged our child. In Zen Center, we hadn't thought of these things because we were so busy, what with manifesting the dharma and the constant power struggles with other Zen students and all.

Finally, one client suggested that we could address our problems by making up a five-year plan and a ten-year plan. These plans would enable us to decide how to achieve financial security and evaluate our progress over time. We agreed that seemed the wise thing to do. Because we wanted to give the plan making a great deal of respect and attention, and make its creation a kind of celebration of our maturity and sobriety, we decided to devote a whole Sunday to it. We would take a long bike ride along the Embarcadero and end up in one of those cute little cafés in Ghirardeli Square. There we would sit and make up our five- and ten-year plans, accompanied by espresso and bread and cheese.

The Sunday we had chosen to devote to our future turned out to be a shimmeringly beautiful San Francisco day: warm but not hot, with enough breeze to caress our cheeks. I stuffed the back-pack with pencils and yellow legal pads, and we climbed on our bikes early in the morning and headed south of Market Street to ride along the wharf down to Ghirardeli Square. We took our time, meandering among the piers and buildings. We stopped to watch a huge ship come in and to browse among the items at a sidewalk sale. It was an exquisite day, with the rippling waves of the bay glistening in the sunlight. By the time we got to Ghirardeli Square, I was very relaxed and expansive, my legs warm and feeling sturdy from all the pedaling, my cheeks rosy from the sun. I was very happy.

We got a table and ordered our cappuccinos, plus a big plate of cheese, sourdough bread, grapes, and pears. "Incredible day," I said to my husband. He agreed. We sat there without speaking for a few moments, cherishing our last taste of languid pleasure before we shifted to our task. I sat for many minutes, waiting to be infused by my usual enthusiasm for organizational work, especially in the service of our futures. Instead, I felt unwilling to shake off my deep contentment. I waited for that feeling to pass, for restlessness to impel me to take up the task, but the resistance got stronger. What's going on? I thought. We should get on with this; we have a lot to do. But increasing certainty was forming in my stomach . . . that this task actually never had anything to do with us in the first place. As we sat under an umbrella, sipping milk and coffee and eating fruit, the buzz of street performers and tourists all around us, I suddenly understood that my real five- and ten-year plans had coalesced during the bike ride. I knew exactly what I wanted to do for the rest of my life.

For the next five years and the next ten years, I wanted to practice meditation and deepen my relationships and advise other people in pain and deeply live all the moments of my life to which I could become awake, just as I had done for the last fifteen years. Most important, I wanted to continue to allow the same intuition that was making this clear to me now to continue to guide my life. And so I finally understood the frantic discomfort of the last few months, how pulled off center I had become from listening to the advice of people who approached their lives in a very precise and rational way. I had originally thought my lack of planning was sloppy, mindless, but at that moment in that café in Ghirardeli Square, I realized that it was not heedless at all; it was actually a value of mine to leave plenty of room for the unconscious to arise and direct my actions.

We put our yellow legal pads away in the backpack, drank our cappuccinos, and rode home through the throng of tourists. I felt as if I had come home after a very long and unpleasant journey far away. We were back under our banners of truth. After some months of taking on other people's views, we had settled back upon our own values. It was great to return.

Before you interpret this story as a putdown of approaching your life rationally and investing your money for your and your children's futures, let me make it very clear that I don't consider financial planning to be inappropriate or "unspiritual" in the least. I think for Tony and me at that time, it generated a frantic feeling to be made suddenly aware of so many factors we had never before considered. As a matter of fact, over the years, we have begun contributing to an IRA and handed over the whole of a small inheritance to a professional financial planner in order to establish some financial security for ourselves. Again, taking care of what needs to be taken care of is part of an engaged life, and yet we must understand that our best efforts to protect ourselves may avail us nothing. There must be room for the unexpected, for it will usually happen. No reasonable plan for our future will box us in and leave us no options, nor will any such plan guarantee our future, but of course, we take an umbrella in case of rain.

One Saturday morning at the San Francisco Zen Center, I told the story about our bike ride to Ghirardeli Square as part of a lecture about trusting your own inherent wisdom. Afterward, several people gathered to ask me questions that had arisen for them during my talk. Sure enough, some of them asked anxiously whether I had implied that financial planning was too premeditated to include in a spiritual practice. I replied very positively that not only was providing for your old age a responsibility you should acknowledge but that it could even be considered a kindness to your friends and relatives. The danger, I declared, lay in looking beyond your current plan, in expecting a secure future to materialize because of your efforts to make it so. I was remembering Katagiri-roshi's admonition that "As long as you are a human being, you are right in the middle of the situation of not understanding anything because life is vast, because it is the truth."

One woman was struggling to grasp the idea of simultaneously planning for the future and not expecting anything to come of it. I couldn't manage to say anything that could help her see the distinction between planning for the future and having expectations for the possible results of those plans. Suddenly a gray-bearded man interrupted and said that in his youth, he had been very concerned about his comfort in his old age and had made it a priority to invest a great deal of money in his future security. He and his wife had in fact retired some years ago in a beautiful house on the East Coast with no financial worries.

"But then the unexpected happened," he said, his face lighting with obvious amusement. "I decided I was gay, I gave my wife the house, and I moved to San Francisco virtually penniless."

We all roared our appreciation. The questioning woman immediately understood. It was a great example of Katagiri's statement, "The point you have to know is that you are right in the situation of not understanding anything." Katagiri continues: "Nowhere to go, no directions, no way to know what it is and if you try to know, this is already a detour. Just do your best to take care of here and now with true heart. . . . Being present right now, right here, with wholeheartedness, is completely beyond your speculation."

When everything is beyond your speculation, there's nothing else you can do but take care of what's right in front of you right now. This is trusting in the connection you feel to your own activity rather than to any results of it. Not that you don't want results, not that you don't care about your future security, but right here in this moment, you engage with your life because you are alive and crave to be connected to everything. Just because you are alive, just because you are a human being, you raise your banner of truth wherever you are, without anticipating any result or expecting that you will be able to control something through the raising of your banner. The control is something extra. Just to do something without any expectation is enough. You do it because it is there to be done. Food to cook, dishes to wash, children to nourish, money to buy what you need and anything extra to invest and anything beyond that to give away. You can do all these things without anticipating any results. In fact, if you try washing the dishes fully present for the motions you are making and the sensations you are feeling as the hot, sudsy water spills over your fingers, revealing the pattern of your china, you may find that's enough. The clean sink at the end is icing on the cake.

5

ECSTASY

The Pleasure That Refreshes

❧ ❧

EXPERIENCING ecstasy from time to time is very important for our general health and well-being. By ecstasy, I mean that timeless, boundless feeling we have whenever we lose our ability to assign more value to one thing than another, to make judgments between this and that, to rate one thing or person or experience higher than another. The critical mind that oppresses us all the time is gone. Everything we encounter is just itself, not more worthwhile than anything else. We're completely immersed in our activity and surroundings; we're taking it all in, every wondrous detail. Our discriminating mind is gone, taking with it all differences in the values of everything we're aware of. Now as we look around us, everything we sense and feel is just as fascinating and beautiful as every other thing we sense and feel. Everything has equal value. That's ecstasy.

We all need to get out from under our critical, judgmental thoughts from time to time and enjoy the freedom of being able to look at things with fresh eyes, with a view unencumbered by our usual opinions. What a flush of relief and refreshment! Thus, it becomes important to notice this experience when it happens to us spontaneously and also to actively cultivate it—that is, to set up situations in which it may occur.

We hear the word *ecstasy* a lot in connection with religious or spiritual matters or, more recently, in connection with what are called "peak experiences," brought on by psychedelic drugs or

mind-expanding exercises that induce a sense of boundary disso-
lution. Our usual unconscious or vaguely uncomfortable feeling
of being separated or alienated from the people and things
around us is suddenly dissolved, and we feel at one with everything. What being "at one with everything" actually means is that
we no longer perceive ourselves as more or less important than,
and therefore separate from, everything else. Usually, we have a
vertical value system with ourselves at the top and our friends
and concerns in descending order. When our boundaries have
dissolved, our value system is suddenly horizontal, completely inclusive. Everything we perceive has the same high value. Our experience has an immediacy, an intensity, that is missing from
a mind that assigns relative value to things according to their
usefulness or beauty. This is indeed an ecstatic feeling, and
having that feeling tends to make us very loving, generous, and
expansive.

Ecstasy is an important kind of pleasure because it challenges
our ingrained habit of thinking of ourselves as a separate entity
forced to satisfy our needs in a not-always-safe "outside world."
As soon as we make the distinction between self and other, we
assign a higher or lower value to our self compared to everything
else. How we perceive the "outside world" is very dependent on
what our agenda is, what we need from the world, what out there
we wish to avoid. It can be educational, not to mention exhila-
rating, to have the boundaries between "us" and "the world"
dissolved.

What triggers the feeling of ecstasy is different for each of us.
Many of us have this feeling when listening to music. Our cares
fall away; our critical judgment disappears, and we are carried
out of our everyday concerns on a stream of sound. My husband,
who works all day with homeless people on the street and with
an often unresponsive bureaucracy, gets pretty cranky if he
doesn't have a chance to go into his room every evening, choose
a CD, and relax on his couch, totally immersed in the music. No
coincidence that much of his collection is blues music of all
kinds. He lies there and lets someone with great skill express the
pain and inevitable despair of his efforts to assuage others' suffer-

ing. Sometimes, looking in on him, I can actually see the guitar chords washing over his chest, releasing the day's accumulation of suffering.

A good friend of mine feels that way about chanting the *Metta-sutta*, the sutra of loving-kindness. (His favorite version is in Jack Kornfield's *A Path with Heart*.) He is a kind person beset with troubles and anxieties. A caring man who is very considerate of other people, he is often distressed by the way others treat him. He expects other people to have the same high standards in interpersonal contact that he does. The little wounds caused by these offenses tend to fester in him until he feels embittered, which of course he hates, and then he feels even more resentful that people don't treat him as well as he expects. This is a cycle that can make him quite ill. Fortunately, he discovered *Metta*. There is something about chanting with his full attention on wishing himself, all his loved ones, and even his enemies safety, health, peace, ease, and happiness that completely dissolves his sense of isolation and pain. After some time of chanting this *sutta*, he feels expansive and open to everything, no longer preoccupied with the injustices done him by insensitive people.

A woman I know reports that she is sometimes spontaneously struck as she's walking down the street by a sudden perception of wholeness that includes her own self and everything around her: the buildings, the cars, the people. It's all just a great, vast mosaic full of color and sound and unsurpassed beauty. Everything simply fits together. There's no ugly, no extraneous, no offensive. Ordinarily when we walk down a city street, we make automatic judgments about the aesthetic merits of one building over another and the attractiveness of the people we see; we recoil at the obvious suffering of the homeless; we think our usual thoughts about the sterility of concrete, the pollution of cars, whatever. We're caught up in the relative world, automatically assigning value to everything we perceive. This woman finds herself temporarily free of all that, able to perceive the integrity of the urban world around her, a place where everything is just *there*. No blame, no fault. She says the experience refreshes her for days.

In stress-reduction classes, I ask students to sit and focus the mind on the information coming in from the senses: sounds, sights, smells, tastes, the sense of other people in the room, and sensations on the skin caused by clothes, hair, jewelry, breeze. People's reactions vary. Some immediately jump from simply perceiving these feelings into judgments about them, whether they are pleasant or unpleasant. Others get a break from judgment; there is a gap between their perception and the rating of it in terms of pleasure. These people report the meditation as "transporting," "energizing," or "relaxing." The feeling I call ecstasy has interrupted the flow of their goal-oriented, self-centered thoughts and allowed them a respite, some moments of peace before they return to the constant natter of judging mind.

My favorite, most reliable form of ecstasy is white-water river rafting. No matter how bound up I am in my arthritic pain, or preoccupied in my work, I am taken out of my ordinary plodding and anxiety-ridden consciousness by river rafting. In fact, I plan several trips well ahead of time just so I will be pulled out of my goal-directed activity later when I would not choose to change my focus. I see a trip coming up in my appointment book, and it's inviolable. I'll drop everything and go. Although I often take five-day, weeklong, or ten-day trips to rivers in other western states, I most frequently just drive up to the nearby American River north of Sacramento for a day trip. You have to be there by ten in the morning, so the night before, I'm assembling piles of equipment.

The enjoyment, if not the loss of my critical mind, starts right away while I'm loading the car. I'm already lighthearted just from the anticipation of connecting with the boundless. Tevas, plastic shorts, bathing suit, a change of clothes, blue-and-purple life jacket (I got my own early on because I look terrible in orange, which is the color of the standard-issue life jackets handed out by rafting companies). Early in the morning on the day of the trip, I start the car in San Francisco's dense fog, turning on the wipers to clear the condensed droplets from the windshield. Because it's so early, I'm virtually alone on the road. In no time, I cross the usually congested Bay Bridge, a structure of great majesty when you aren't cursing the traffic. The fog will give way to brilliant sunshine as I drive farther inland, but it won't be uncomfortably hot for hours.

I've brought several tapes for the car stereo, and this is unusual in itself for me: listening to music for a long, uninterrupted period of time. My ordinary life doesn't allow this. At home, my work and family life demand constant interaction with other people. When I have any free time, I tend to want it quiet, so I can just receive incidental sounds: the birds, schoolchildren's voices as they pass by, the internal noises of the apartment building. But music is perfect for driving, and I love it. The rock 'n' roll I play loud; the blues I play soft to enjoy the mood.

By the time I reach the Motherlode put-in place, I'm very mellow indeed. Not quite nonjudgmental, however. I greet my fellow rafters as they arrive and have a strong, unvoiced opinion about every one: how attractive, how bright, how friendly, how appropriate or absurd I find their attire, how ridiculous they look in those shorts, or how I envy their silhouette in a wet suit. Oh, God, I'm thinking, please don't let me get *that* person in my boat. What was she thinking, dressing like that with that body? Or what a droll wit that person has; I hope we're in the same boat! The guides meander among us, checking our life jackets. I have my favorites among them, too, and I'm chatting them up, angling to be chosen by this one, hoping my admiration is returned sufficiently to be included in his or her raft for the day. I'm doing my usual social thing, meting out judgments and preferences right and left.

Eventually the rafts are ready, and the guides assign us to various ones. I'm either happy or petulant about my assigned raftmates. We push off from the bank, and I'm grumbling to myself, "Stuck with this dimwit! I have to look at that stupid T-shirt for hours!" I notice a beer can in the water. "What idiot left that there in such a beautiful place as this! People are pigs!" And so on down the river.

But then we hit that first rapid. All my mental talk stops as the adrenaline hits my bloodstream. We get through it and drift again in calm water. After the splashing and the yelling and the fear and the delight, I'm free. No more judgments, no more oppressive criticism. My raftmate is the perfect companion for this adventure. If I see any more beer cans or plastic in the water, I regard it as part of the scenery: beautiful the way the sun glints off the metal! My whole world is sun and cold water and the stretch of spandex across my belly. The peanut butter sandwiches at lunch are the most welcome, delicious nourishment I have ever taken. My companions are the pinnacle of wit and courage. No more comparisons. These moments are the only moments that have ever existed. Such experiences have put my rheumatoid arthritis into remission for as long as several months. More than a refreshment to me—though that would certainly be reward enough—ecstasy is an essential part of my healing.

We can take an ecstatic experience like this back into our ordinary lives. Even after it's over and our boundaries and judgments have returned, just the fact that we had such an experience frees us up. We may never again be oppressed by our critical, negative mind in exactly the same way. What ecstasy offers us is the chance to have a tiny bit of detachment from our usual separate-making mind; maybe we'll never believe that mind totally, completely, again. The reason we might take the trouble to cultivate ecstasy and build it into our lives occasionally is because it rejuvenates us so thoroughly. It's as if we were starting our lives all over again from a different perspective.

But as wonderful and renewing as ecstasy is, of course, we don't want to cling to it. We would be subverting the experience and changing its very nature as a perception of completeness by starting to chase it, to prefer it to the other mind states we experience in our lives. Yet it's such a powerful, lucent experience, it's hard to let it pass of its own accord. We feel as if we have actually been *sane* for some short period of time and now must go back to some demented rendition of reality. It requires some mental stability, some appreciation for ordinary life as it is, to let ecstasy fade and return again to our separate world of the self and its high-maintenance demands. Our cultivation of ecstasy must be disinterested; we refresh and revive ourselves with it periodically just as we enjoy sitting down with an iced drink after carrying a heavy load. We must be willing to let ecstasy come and go, or we will turn a great pleasure into a great prison.

THE TRAP OF CHASING AFTER ECSTASY

If ecstasy is just another kind of pleasure you chase after, like praise or sexual relief, it cannot retain its essential character as the perception of the completeness of things as they are. It is this perception, that nothing has more value than anything else, that brings on the feeling of immersion that you love so about this state of mind. When you chase after a particular state of mind, you as an entity are still the reference point, and you set yourself up to pursue ecstasy as an object separate from you. This is the problem noted in Chapter 1 when Trungpa described the realm of the gods. You see yourself and your state of mind as two different things.

If you get so attached to this golden state of mind that your ordinary life seems hopelessly depressing by comparison, then it's as if you've fallen into a thicket of "entangling vines," as Hsueh Tou calls this mesmerized state in the *Blue Cliff Record* verse cited in Chapter 1. You're so preoccupied with achieving another state of mind, you lose your ability to be present in your actual life, and you get impatient with the suffering of other people. Even while you're in ecstasy, you subvert and change it into a state of suffering because you're worried that you might get knocked out of this wonderful state of mind. Thus, your attachment to bliss destroys not only your participation in your ordinary life but the quality of the bliss itself.

On the other hand, if you live your life in such a thoroughgoing way that you are always immersing yourself in each activity, one after the other without reluctance, there's no extra feeling of you and it. It's not you relating to something you call bliss. There's just connection, awareness of the whole; that's the only thing there is. When you are deeply immersed in the activities of your life, these experiences may be frequent, but you won't notice them. As soon as you step back to perceive yourself having

an "ecstatic" moment, there's you and the moment again, subject and object. These thoughts are extra; a full, rich life of immersion is enough.

In a dharma lecture, Reb Anderson, the practice leader of
Green Gulch, says:

> Being willing to give up great [joy] and to become involved
> again in particular thoughts is compassion. In this way we
> knowingly and willingly re-enter the world of confusion and
> suffering. We feel connection with all the different varieties of
> suffering. Our body interacts fearlessly with all forms of suffer-
> ing. Whenever our mind is completely open and we are not
> controlling what we are exposed to, the body and mind can sit
> still in the heart of all suffering beings. That is all we have to
> do. Everything else will take care of itself.

I think it possible that this kind of immersion in suffering may
produce a feeling of wholeness that is indistinguishable from
bliss.

6

NURTURING RELATIONSHIPS

❧ ❦

A s human beings, we are always in relationship to something. Our minds naturally divide the world into "I" and "thou," thereby creating an "other" to whom to relate. I don't think this mental tendency is necessarily a bad thing that we should strive to stop doing in order to make the world a more coherent place. Instead, I think our efforts might be more usefully directed toward discovering our interconnectedness with all people and things and regarding all of the endless variation we experience in the world as the elements of our spiritual life. No relationship to anything can be excluded from our spiritual life.

Those who have chosen to live a focused spiritual life within a community of like-minded people understand that our relationships to our teachers and fellow practitioners are important. But what such devotees often tend to overlook is the towering importance of our relations with our spouses, our children, our parents, our coworkers, even our relations with the clerks in the stores where we shop, the people we pass on the street, the toll collector on the bridge, the beggar pleading to wash our car windows, the person auditing us for the IRS, the driver who cuts us off on the freeway—or the driver we cut off. Everybody counts! None of these relationships is more sacred than any other; all these people are our teachers. Each encounter is an opportunity to receive the teaching of compassion, to be suddenly struck with the interconnectedness of all life. If we practice encounter in such a thoroughgoing way, compassion naturally develops.

What is important to us if we are overwhelmed by pain or

stress is to avail ourselves of the powerful healing and comfort afforded by close relationships with other people. Unfortunately, not just any relationship, such as many of those we already have, will do. When we are already exhausted, drained from feeling chronic pain ourselves or from the burden of caring for someone very ill, we need to have relationships that nurture and sustain us rather than those that further drain us. If we live in chronic pain or with a stressful situation that we cannot change, it is crucial to be surrounded by kind and pleasing companions, at least one or two. It's not that our nurturers must be skilled at nursing or wise counselors; they only need to be supportive and considerate of us. Sometimes when we are so miserable that it is nearly unendurable, the only thing that helps is having someone to silently hold our hand while we go to hell.

I learned the importance of being nurtured by other people for the first time as I began to slowly recover from a phase of my illness in which I was bedridden. As I interacted with people other than my immediate caretakers again, I was very surprised to notice how dramatically my social interactions affected my energy level. Before I got sick, I had led a very unexamined social life. People asked me to accompany them to events, and I usually said yes. Because I had lots of energy, I didn't have to worry that any particular person or event would compromise me. But after I was sick, I saw that particular persons had a tremendous impact on my well-being. Some people were so easy to be around that my energy level actually went up in their company, as if as long as they were present I were being carried in a hammock or one of those big Hawaiian wicker chairs that look like thrones. When these people came to make my dinner or wash my hair, I wanted them to stay with me forever. I actually felt better physically when they were around, as if they cushioned something for me.

But there were also people whose company was actually dangerous for me. When they came to help, I would always feel more tired after they left than before they came. They seemed to take something away from the little I had. Sometimes after spending time with such a person, I would be so drained that I had to stay in bed the whole next day. I soon understood that I had to start being careful about whom I spent time with. The problem was that I couldn't tell beforehand who would help or hurt me. I tried very hard to see what it was about a person that made him or her an energy-drainer or an energy-giver, but I just couldn't tell. I seemed to be too distracted by how a person looked, what he was wearing, how witty she was, and so on, none of which appeared to be relevant.

Finally I hit upon the idea of using my breathing as my guide. If I was in the company of someone who expanded my breathing, who made my breaths long and deep, I stayed with that person for as long as he or she would tolerate my company. Relaxed and energized, I could hardly bear to leave. Whenever someone inhibited my breathing, caused it to be shallow or irregular, I quickly made my excuses to leave, thereby averting collapse later. This practice worked so well, I was sorry to give it up as I got more robust, though I had to because my social relationships became much more complicated.

We often find ourselves working with or married to people who periodically inhibit our breathing. I think one of the most difficult relationships to maintain at a nurturing level, besides blood family (a special challenge of its own), is the intimate relationship with a spouse, a lover. Sometimes a clergyman will be a deeply religious individual, a wonderful role model for everyone, an inspiration to parishioners to shape their everyday life from their religious beliefs. Mindful in every task, kind to every sentient being, he is loved and respected by all. But his wife has a different picture. She can't get him to pay attention to her, to be even a passable husband in terms of valuing their relationship. He's too busy writing sermons and counseling his flock. By the time he gets home, he's too exhausted to treat her like the unique and wondrous sentient being she is, deserving of the same respect he gives each one of his parishioners. Instead, he'd like a little downtime from consciousness. Why is this scenario so common? Why are our mates often the last people to benefit from our rigorous and sincere practice of self-awareness and compassion?

I think part of the problem is how we choose our mates and

why we want to have mates. For starters, we need helpmeets to
share the economic and time concerns of raising a family in a
competitive society in which the goods to which we all feel entitled are relatively scarce. We also need partners to make us feel
secure, to assure us that we are wonderful because there's a short-
age of other people who will. Such reassuring lovers and friends
help keep our fears at bay. They provide the attention, validation,
protection, and drama we all need to keep ourselves going. But
when we begin to mature as human beings, to develop the aspect
of ourselves that takes an inclusive view of "other," we cultivate
attitudes that enable us to support life in general. Individual relationships are just one aspect of opening the heart to all that is.
To truly support somebody means that we offer him or her whatever we can and expect nothing in return. This doesn't mean
that we don't have a parallel sensibility that is alert to the give-
and-take inherent in any functioning relationship; I'm talking
fundamental attitude here. I'm talking about wishing for the
well-being of our mate so sincerely that we could be like the wife
dying of cancer who tries to arrange a relationship for her husband with one of her friends in order for him to be comforted
after her death.

Ongoing and long-term relationships are our best source of
growth as well as comfort, especially relationships with people
who are willing to roll up their sleeves and get into their own and
our respective muck about what is and what should be. In early
Buddhism, celibacy was challenged by teachers who argued that
although a monk might be able to fool the other monks into
thinking he had attained great, virtuous states of mind through
his meditation, no monk could fool his wife. If our friends are
willing to be candid about their responses to our words and actions, we can see what our opinions, judgments, projections, and
thoughts really are, free of the ideals to which we cling. If we
observe our thoughts and actions closely with some degree of
detachment when we're with our blood relatives, we can see
where we're stuck and what we're holding on to. Blood relatives
are great for inadvertently pointing out to us where our buttons
are and pushing them. After all, they're the ones who installed

the buttons in the first place. Thus, we have a great chance to learn and grow in their company. So all our relationships are indispensable to our personal development if we are able to follow our interactions with curiosity.

When we begin to understand what our true motives are with regard to other people, we realize that we are blinded to others' points of view by our own opinions and agendas. We are appalled to discover our unkind and selfish thoughts about other people and our preoccupation with how they might be manipulated to serve our purposes. Once we have discovered our own supreme importance in our world, we might wonder how any of us manages to have any relationships at all that span this self-absorption, but our ego-centeredness is not the only game in town. It's just very powerful. We also have altruistic and empathetic parts of us that yearn to know and protect others. But we must make conscious how terrible we think someone is or how terrible we think we are, what we want, what we expect, what we think is right or superior, because all these thoughts are the basic ground for every encounter. When we investigate this ground and come to know it well, we can open ourselves to others without fear.

From personal experience, I would have to say that it's very difficult to be intimate with things and people when our views are primary and fixed. Often we can't see what is really there because we're too busy asserting ourselves and our views. And it's really, really hard to get breathing space from our opinions, to catch a glimpse of situations without that overlay, for more than moments at a time. An interesting game I play with myself is to watch my views go by while I'm reading the newspaper. The fun comes from the fact that stories in the newspaper evoke all kinds of opinions in me that I'm not ordinarily aware that I have. So I watch myself reconcile the outcomes of the news stories to my own personal worldview. For instance, I really like when people shoot cacti and the cacti fall over on them and crush them. That supports my worldview that even plants can enjoy some kind of justice. I also like to read that somebody had a really good idea and got rich from it in his or her later years, like Ray Kroc, the founder of McDonald's. Or that some grandmother hit a drug dealer over the head with her frying pan, scaring him so badly that he ran away. I don't like to read that the dealer shot her instead.

I like to read that someone saved a person of a different race from a fire. Or that some simple idea like the Midnight Basketball League can make the crime statistics go down. I like reading about events like that because they support my worldview that there is such a thing as justice, that good is rewarded materially and bad punished, that maybe the universe itself is benevolent, and that virtue and cooperation are the natural state of the universe, whereas ignorance and harming are aberrant behavior with limited effect. So of course, I really hate reading that somebody who tried to save someone else from being mugged is shot and killed himself. Or that companies whose corporate executives lay off workers and refuse to extend benefits make lots more money than businesses that treat their workers as if they were an important and indispensable part of the business. Or that a woman who spent her adult life trying to improve the conditions of ghetto children is shot and killed by a random bullet. This confuses and diminishes me. I want the world to be more than a benevolent place: I want it to be a comprehensible place in which events make sense to me personally.

But sometimes when I start to read the newspaper, I discover that, for whatever reason, I don't have all my views in place just then. I'm unexpectedly open. When that happens, what I feel are just the emotions engendered by the story: admiration for the brave or clever person, sorrow at losing someone who was making my world more humane. It feels like a relief when I'm not always trying to reconcile reality to my ideas of right and wrong. It's ironic that I should prefer it that way because that way is actually the most painful. I feel what it's like to be deprived of a brave and kind person; feel what it's like to have less of the rain forest, less of a live earth; feel the fear that I could be at the mercy of murderers myself, like people in Bosnia or Rwanda. Sometimes I am even made to wonder what could turn me into a murderer. Seeing someone viciously hurt my child? So why would I prefer experiencing these often unpleasant feelings to struggling mentally for a few moments to reconcile everything to my worldview? Because of the connection. The feeling that when the earth heaves, I heave. When someone is tortured, I am tortured. When someone is hurt, I hurt. When someone is brave, I, too, would be brave in his or her place. It is very strangely comforting at the same time that it is painful.

At any given time, we have a viewpoint or stance about life; we include some things, exclude others. If we're sincerely attempting to free ourselves of the tyranny of our stances in order to glimpse a world unconditioned by our prejudices, our attempts themselves will shake up those viewpoints. As we begin to question our viewpoints, we may feel irritated, upset, as we try to reconcile our views with a broader perspective. We may even feel as if we're losing our self, our identity as a New Ager, a left-winger, a Democrat, a reasonable person, whatever. Finally we become willing to experience our suffering as beings interconnected with other beings. When we actually feel our feelings and our connectedness, our worldview shifts radically to include more and more situations and people. Each time we do this, each time we go into the suffering and let it be, our vision of life enlarges. So it interests me to see ways in which my views prevent this connection and make me feel separate—not just separate as an individual but estranged.

Recently I went down to Zen Mountain Center, a summer resort run by the San Francisco Zen Center. First step out of the shuttle, I happened to meet a woman who is always trying to talk to me in a hearty manner whenever we run into each other. I usually try to avoid her because I regard whatever conversation we have as trivial and about topics that don't interest me. So naturally I'd rather spend my rare and therefore precious social time talking with people I regard as more interesting, whom I come away from feeling as if I made a connection. But in this instance, a chat with her was unavoidable; there was no place to escape to short of climbing a steep hillside to get out of the Tassajara valley. She captured me, I was hers, and we had a conversation. It was boring, we parted finally, and I complained later to a close friend that I had been taken prisoner and benumbed. She laughed at my description.

But then the very next day, my close friend and I got into a disagreement and had to work out some hurt feelings between us. Practiced in this art from years of intimacy with each other, we spoke very candidly, one to the other, describing carefully how we each had been hurt by what we thought was being said. Because of how focused we were on our interaction, I felt extremely engaged with my friend and close to her. I came away from this conversation energized by the connection my good friend and I had made with each other. With no small amount of self-satisfaction, I saw our hurt feelings as the compost that nurtures intimacy. Suddenly I started thinking about my boring talk with the other woman. What a contrast. It occurred to me in thinking about how present I was with my friend, how careful to check my own feelings and to consider hers, was it possible I had some responsibility for the lack of connection between me and the other woman?

The next time I ran into the boring woman, I adjusted my perception to see whether it made any difference. First, I elevated her to the same status as my friend and myself: an endlessly fascinating and worthwhile human being. Then I made the same effort to be present with her as I had with my friend. Now that she was a human being instead of a nitwit, it wasn't even that hard. When she said things I didn't follow, I noticed my tendency to dismiss her views, but I kept asking her what she meant until I understood what she was trying to say. When she expressed feelings I didn't share, I told her my feelings as well. She totally met me; there was no holding back on her part. We had a lively conversation. I came away deeply impressed with how much responsibility had been mine in making our talks boring. In my judgment of her, I had been coming to rest in the alienating rather than the connecting points in our conversation. That relationship changed from energy-draining to energy-giving because I changed my participation in it.

Recently I was greatly shocked to discover how views that I was kind of embarrassed about, but never bothered to reexamine, had really hurt my favorite nephew's new wife. For years, I have turned down invitations to the Passover Seder meal, a springtime ritual that celebrates the passage of the Jews from slavery in Egypt through the parted Red Sea to freedom. Not that I didn't think Jews should celebrate their liberation, of course, but I was offended by the idea of a vengeful God smiting the firstborn children of Egypt when Pharaoh refused to free the Hebrews. Those firstborn children, many of them infants and toddlers, hadn't hurt anybody. So last year when my nephew and his new wife, she a practicing Jew, asked me to come to their Seder, I chose not to go.

But this year, my nephew's mother, Laura, my sister-in-law, with whom I am quite close, called me. She said she needed to talk to me about something troubling. I immediately put myself at her disposal; I couldn't imagine what trouble could have arisen between us. Then she said, "I hope you are planning to accept Danny and Elaine's Seder invitation this year because they were very hurt last year when you didn't go." Genuinely surprised, I said, "Really?" Laura went on to tell me that Danny and his new wife felt that I was actually anti-Semitic and were afraid that it might cause a rift in the family because they intended to raise the baby they were expecting as a Jew.

I was horrified to think I had so callously hurt them by such an offhand action on my part. It hadn't occurred to me they would think anything of it. In fact, I hadn't actually said why I wasn't going; I just declined. Why did they think I was anti-Semitic? Then, with mounting shame, I recalled the Jewish jokes I had told Elaine, thinking she wouldn't take offense because I was born half-Jewish myself. Didn't that give me the right to make jokes if we were both Jewish? I suddenly felt my cheeks get hot as I held the phone receiver. I was deeply and painfully ashamed. I was aware of some distaste I felt toward the Jewish religion (as opposed to actual Jewish people) because of the patriarchy and hypocrisy that I associated with Judaism in my own childhood, but I never took the trouble to revisit these views since I had not been in a situation that touched on them—that is, in the company of practicing Jews—for many, many years. I realized on the phone with Laura that I had thought of my anti-Judaism (not anti-Semitism) as harmless because it was dormant, never evoked. But here it was, spread out before me, and not a pretty sight.

Contrite, I thanked Laura very much for telling me all this and immediately called up Danny and Elaine. Elaine herself answered the phone, and I apologized for my attitude, my jokes, and how unwelcome all this must have been to her in her new family and said how sorry I was for the hurt I had caused her. I ended by saying that if she would extend me an invitation to their Seder this year, I would be honored to come. She actually cried tears of relief on the phone. I cringed at the sound of her relief because I knew it was in proportion to how much worry I had caused her.

Then I called Laura back and told her I had apologized and was going to the Seder, and so was my husband. Laura was happy. She remarked, "It's so good you did that. After all, they have a baby coming and a new house, and they should have the family all together this Seder for support." I agreed. Then just before we hung up, Laura, who is a very politically correct, globally concerned person, asked me, "By the way, what was it you so objected to about a Seder that you wouldn't go last year?" I said, "It's all the smiting. The Hebrew God killed all the firstborn Egyptian children because the pharaoh wouldn't let the Israelites go. I think that's why it's called Passover, because the angel of death passed over the Jewish homes while killing all the Egyptian firstborn." "Really?!" Laura exclaimed. "I never thought of it that way! That's terrible! I'm not going to the Seder unless they let me say a prayer for the firstborn Egyptian children!" I got off the phone feeling vaguely surreal because of the uncomfortable thought that rather than healing a breach for Danny and Elaine's sake, Laura and I had just swapped views.

Sure enough, Danny called soon after. Not realizing that Laura and I had already talked, he pleaded with me to call his mother and try to soothe her. He said she had read him a prayer for the dead Egyptian children, and it sounded to him like an anti-Semitic diatribe that he didn't think his wife could tolerate.

When he had told his mother she couldn't read her prayer for the Egyptian children, she accused him of not allowing other points of view, a high crime in this particular family, at the Seder. "It's *our* Seder," he wailed to me.

Guilt-struck, I called Laura, and together we worked out a prayer that was basically for all children everywhere. I called Danny; it was acceptable. Whew! All was well at last. I must tell you it didn't escape me how ironic it was for me, the accused anti-Semite, to be playing peacemaker here. Finally, after peace seemed assured, all this struck me as very funny, an example of what can happen when you hold your own views as more important than your relationships to other people.

Because I thought it was such a humorous story, and it had seemed to work out so well, I told it to a friend who was raised Orthodox Jewish. Instead of laughing, her voice took on a warning tone. "Well, I hope the Seder is not going to be so strictly Orthodox that only men will be allowed to say the prayers," she told me. New fears arose. I thought, Oh, no, if Laura can't read her prayer, the whole controversy will erupt right there, and the family will be sundered, if not forever, at least at a very sensitive time.

My husband and I drove to the Seder as if going to a funeral. I thought we might be: the death of our so far extraordinarily good family relations between nephew, new wife, sister-in-law, brother, and so forth. But as it turned out, we needn't have worried. Elaine had astutely and skillfully taken care of the whole thing. She had us all take turns reading from the Seder prayer book; plus she had eliminated any reference to smiting anyone and had even selected an admonishment in the prayer book not to gloat over the bodies of the vanquished enemy. Laura said her brief prayer for all children at the end. Full of Mogen David wine, hard-boiled egg, apple, and the reassuring warmth of goodwill among kinfolk, I nodded off. It was a very successful Seder, sure to become a tradition in our newly constellated family.

I left feeling particularly connected to Laura and Elaine, since we all three had voluntarily shifted our views to accommodate the others. So the connection and the difference can exist simultaneously at different levels of us. We are connecting on one level and being disparate on another. None of these connections and differences hinder one another. This is all very rich and complex, many of the lush possibilities of life on view at the same time. Later my brother and I discussed how everyone had participated in making it such a success; we had all shifted our views enough so that they included everyone else, a triumph of communality. I did add wickedly, "If the Egyptians ever find out about this Seder thing, they're going to be really mad." "They did and they are," my brother said. He had the last word.

I think any kind of felt connection is nurturing, regardless of whether there is a relationship container. Some of the most energizing encounters I have ever had have been brief ones on the street with strangers. Once I had a very lively exchange with a Porsche driver who pulled up alongside me on my bike at a stoplight. When the light changed, he started to turn right, I started going straight, and he knocked me over. Furious, I yelled, "Why don't you watch where you're going?!" He got out of his car, stuck his face in mine, and said, "Why don't *you* watch where *you're* going?!" I said, "Fuck you!" He said, "Fuck you!" Then I said, "Fuck you!" again, and he said, "Fuck you!" again, and we both said it faster and faster several more times until we both dissolved in laughter. Then we wished each other a good day and went on our ways.

I've never forgotten that suddenly intimate connection with a stranger who had nearly injured me. I don't know what changed it from rancorous to friendly. I remember that during the *fuck-yous*, I began to think it was very funny. We were having a classic urban moment. Maybe I changed it, thinking that. But he certainly was ready to connect rather than stay angry, so he was accessible, too. Maybe I picked the humor up from him; maybe he thought it was funny from the beginning but recognized his responsibility to keep up his end of a street argument in the big city. Who knows? But we were both willing to move toward each other and connect right in the midst of our alienation. Again, the connection and the difference existed simultaneously at different levels of us. We were connecting on one level at the same time that we were contentious on another. Neither hinders the other.

What is this intimacy? Not turning away, not touching; letting someone be, letting yourself be, holding your own space, respecting someone else's. When a panhandler approaches, do you respond from the viewpoint of how you would like your money to be spent or how guilty you feel that you are not as unfortunate, or do you just interact with another human being? You might be aware of your disparate positions in society, your judgment of the other person's situation or behavior, even feel aesthetic distaste, but you can choose, if you want, to come to rest in the connecting points rather than the alienating points in your encounter. There may be nothing to connect on but the experience you have that you and this person are both breath and need. Maybe you're feeling generous and expansive that day; maybe you're in no mood, you say so, and you hurry on. When you resist having a stance or a policy about giving to people on the street that you automatically trot out in every instance, you can respond from your feelings at the moment.

WHORE STORIES

As an urban person, I love the sudden flash of intimacy with strangers. Living in San Francisco, I often say, "And the stranger, the better." For many years before gentrification, the neighborhood in which I live was inhabited mostly by very poor people, drug addicts, and prostitutes. At first, I felt threatened by these people so different from me in style and values, but they were often very friendly. The whores, as they waited to be picked up on the corner, passed the time by striking up conversations with me as I passed, so I gradually became much less standoffish. After my husband became a social worker and actually got some of the "girls" off the street and settled in rooms and drug treatment programs, our corner whores became very protective and sweet toward me as his wife. They often carried heavy packages for me, my arthritis being apparent to all but the most casual observer. I began reciprocating with flowers, herbs, and maternal scoldings whenever anyone tried to sell me hot goods.

One night as I walked the two blocks from my parking space to my home, I saw a large man lurking right in front of my building. I was frightened and also annoyed that what I probably should do was knock at a nearby friend's door, disturb him, and ask him to walk me home. I much preferred just going straight to my door rather than backtracking, so I approached the man very slowly, trying to gauge whether he was a threat to me. Just as I came within several yards of him, both he and I were startled by a terrible screech. The prostitute Sylvia, whom I knew well, charged across the street and confronted him: "Go on now!" she cried, shooing him away with her hand motions. "Don't you dare touch a hair on her head!" He got out of there fast, looking bewildered and unjustly set upon. Sylvia greeted me reassuringly as I raised my key to the lock on my door: "Don't you ever worry about anything while I'm around!" I believed her.

Another time, a priest at Zen Center insisted on walking me home after dark. Sylvia must have been distracted because she didn't catch sight of us until we were at my door. Then she pounced, screeching at my friend as vehemently as she had at the lurking man: "You get away from her!" My priest friend went rigid with fear. As Sylvia crossed the street to where we stood, I whispered teasingly, "Don't make any sudden moves, Tom." After assuring Sylvia I was safe, I introduced her to Tom, who was in the process of recovering from her verbal assault. They had a genial exchange, which I hugely enjoyed.

But I think my favorite street connection story is actually someone else's. On election night in 1992, with Clinton ahead in the Democrats' first real challenge to conservative Republicans in more than a decade, my friend Alice was on her way to her car, which necessitated her stepping her way through a large gathering of prostitutes who were blocking the sidewalk, talking animatedly to each other. Alice is a very serious practitioner and scholar of Zen Buddhism who has taught the interconnectedness of all things for many years in classes and to individual students who consider her their Zen teacher. Also by nature a somewhat reserved person, she thought maybe she should cross the street to avoid this rather raucous gathering. Just as she veered toward the curb, one of the whores caught her sleeve to get her attention. Alice braced for trouble. "We're winning!" cried the girl to Alice. "Our side is winning the election!" She spontaneously embraced Alice, who suddenly saw that the women were gathered around a small radio, listening to the election returns as they came in. Everyone was very excited, and they obviously were including Alice from a feeling of exuberant good-fellowship. Alice felt chagrined. "They connected with me," she told me later. "I had rejected them as whores, as trouble, but they didn't do that kind of separation with me. They wanted to share their excitement."

Connection happens only in this very moment. Only in the present can you feel connected with someone or something. Otherwise, it's abstract, a memory or an intention to be connected. In any particular moment when you are experiencing someone else, when you feel intimacy, it's not exactly that you don't feel separate from him or her, merging as opposed to being yourself, but it's more that it's all there in the mix and none of it hinders any aspect of it. Your ideas of compassion or service to others interfere with actual intimacy with another person. You might relate to your own ideals and projections rather than relating to the person in front of you. If you work at a hospice, you do each thing for its own sake. You clean, you feed, you comfort, you breathe—all for its own sake. If you don't understand the difference between helping someone and doing each thing for its own sake, try to remember a time when someone was helping you with a close eye on how grateful you seemed to be. Or the "helper" appeared vaguely preoccupied, as if he or she were absorbed with the thought of doing a good deed.

When I was very ill and needed help with the simplest activities like washing my hair, I found it draining to be helped by people whom I constantly had to reassure that they were doing enough, doing things the right way, seeing me often enough. They paid much more attention to their ideas of "helping a person in need" than to me personally. How refreshing and soothing it was to be tended to by people who were able to approach me directly, without ideas about what they were doing with me, without using me to define who they were at that moment. This was not a subtle difference to me at the time; it was roaringly blatant. The two approaches produced a dramatically different impact on my energy level. The poison of doing good cannot be overestimated. As Jack Kornfield points out in *A Path with Heart,* "Even the most transcendent visions of spirituality must shine through the here and now and be brought to life in how we walk, eat and love one another."

If you are suffering, the important relationships to you now are those that support the part of you that is vulnerable but struggling to deal realistically with a difficult situation. This is not the time to waste your energy on people who value your effervescence above all or those who feel threatened by your frank assessment of your situation. Assign other people to take care of them. Now you need people who are ready to support the aspect of you that must face catastrophe with courage and truth. Don't be afraid that you appear too needy to such friends. When you settle into your true grief, you are not wearing on people in the way that people are before they face their suffering. I myself have stayed up through the night with suffering people and in the morning felt physically tired but psychically energized. I believe the energy came from being in the presence of someone who had become one with suffering, who was penetrating to the heart of human sorrow. If you can do this, you are encouraging and inspiring to your friends. This is not the stiff-upper-lip behavior of the denier; this is grief and tears and agony, but it's real. This difference is palpable to those who wish to comfort you.

7

MAD AS HELL AND CAN'T TAKE ONE MORE THING

Dealing with the Anger Pain Provokes

❧ ❧

Men are admitted into Heaven not because they have curbed and governed their passions or have no passions but because they have cultivated their understandings. The treasures of Heaven are not negations of passion but realities of intellect from which all the passions emanate uncurbed in their Eternal Glory.

—WILLIAM BLAKE

W HEN we experience great suffering, particularly physical pain that won't go away or a chronically stressful situation that cannot be resolved quickly, we find ourselves on a short fuse. There is just plain not enough of us available to absorb yet another problem, even a relatively minor annoyance, when we are preoccupied with our ongoing pain. A mate's forgetfulness, a child's constant prattle, a traffic jam, a mistake at the bank—and we go ballistic. And then afterward, when we see the shattered look on a loved one's face or the conviction of a public servant that we have lost our minds or the outraged response from the stranger on whom we just vented, we are filled with regret. And concern about our own mental health. How come I'm so jumpy? So irritable? So short-tempered?

The truth is, when we are already pushed to the edge by our

chronic pain, our mother's cancer, our child's failure in school, our company's downsizing, how can we take another blow? When a mixture of fear, anguish, and rage fills our hearts, how can we absorb the petty annoyances that life is full of? Unfortunately, I think our friends, coworkers, and relatives expect us to keep our mouths shut and absorb our pain gracefully—that is, without bothering them. Complaining about our troubles or strenuously objecting to a commonplace annoyance—say, call waiting—may be the last taboo in polite society.

NEGATIONS OF PASSION

In my many years of associating with high-minded people who declare their most honored value to be that of doing no harm to others, I would have to say that the most confusing issue in actualizing such a life is how we handle our anger. I think this confusion comes from many sources. One of them is, of course, the conflicting messages about how to express emotion in our culture, or in our various cultures, since it depends so much on what kind of ethnic or racial background you come from. But another huge source of confusion is our idea of spiritual maturity itself and how we interpret the admonitions of our religious teachers.

Many interpretations of spiritual practice definitely seem to imply that we should be trying to suppress anger altogether. Jesus meekly turns his other cheek rather than strike back. In the *Abhidharma*, one of the oldest texts in Buddhism, anger "has the function of causing oneself not to remain in contact with happiness and serves as a basis for misconduct. Through anger, one does not abide in happiness in this lifetime, and immeasurable suffering is induced in the future. Anger is an impatience and intent to harm that arises when a harmful sentient being, or one's own suffering, or sources of suffering, appear to the mind." The *Abhidharma* also says that the aim of meditation practice is the "domestication of man's [and presumably women's] untamed and unbridled emotive nature." What does that mean, the "domestication of man's untamed and unbridled emotive nature"? Is this acceptable to postmodern Americans at the turn of the twenty-first century? After all we've been through shaking off the Victorians and the Eisenhower era? The "domestication of man's untamed and unbridled emotive nature" indeed.

As a culture, we idealize equanimity, certainly. We think either consciously or unconsciously that a "spiritual" person, or a developmentally mature person, is not supposed to get visibly upset over anything. We have Good identified with mildness, temperance (not too much ice cream, coffee, whatever), nonconfronting (it is a very big deal to many people if someone actually directly tells them that they object to them in some way), and serenity. We expect our religious leaders to be serene and sunny, efficient and helpful, some variant of Mary Poppins or Smokey the Bear.

When we're very upset, we sometimes talk about "getting beyond it," using our spiritual aspirations as a way to step out of what we're feeling. We leap into our "higher selves" very quickly. But I see in myself and others a tendency to do this maybe a tad too quickly, thereby cutting off feeling rather than working through it. Doing this immediately, before grappling with passion, seems a little too knee-jerk to me, more like an unexamined habit pattern than a genuine comfort with, and acceptance of, the feelings that have arisen.

Anita Barrows asks in "The Light of Outrage," "If we leap too quickly into forgiveness and loving-kindness, don't we risk losing an opportunity to correct the imbalance or injustice, to take right action? If we drain the energy from anger by neutralizing it too fast, don't we risk compromising our own vitality?"

Do we confuse "domesticating" or "taming" our anger, as Buddhist texts direct, with repressing our anger? How are we supposed to handle our strong emotions, anyway? Could it be a matter of developing patience and skill with our feelings rather than purging them? And what about equanimity? We hold that as an ideal and admire people who are imperturbable no matter what happens to them. Is this admiration misplaced? Are these people just numb? Should we be waking them up instead of reinforcing their defense mechanisms?

Or do they just not care? Sometimes emotional withdrawal behind a cloak of imperturbability can look like equanimity. Actually there is a profound difference between indifference and equanimity. When you really don't care what happens in a particular situation, by definition you're not emotionally involved. So you're not upset by any turn of events; thus, your response can look to observers like serenity. You simply don't care. In contrast, true equanimity is when you are very involved and care terribly what happens, but although a disadvantageous turn of events might disappoint you, it doesn't knock you off your seat or take away your ability to make clear and conscious choices in the situation. Though emotionally shaken, you will still take on the new circumstances with the same wholeheartedness you brought to the situation when it looked hopeful. This does *not* mean that you don't express your disappointment by a few well-chosen words or a well-aimed kick at a piece of furniture.

If we hold equanimity as the standard, we might think less of our friends or spiritual leaders if their marriages break up or they get cancer or they display temper. Such judgments come out of the notion that someone who is successfully coping with adversity is never perturbed or resentful of his or her misfortune. If we value a stance of serenity as indicative of emotional stability, we may make the mistake of suppressing any feelings that accompany our hardships. Then, in the midst of our adversity, we not only have the trouble of the adversity itself, but we have the added burden of squishing ourselves into a certain emotional stance. Often people who have committed themselves to a spiritual practice overlook the opportunity to express their own individual suffering in favor of feigning an impersonal state of mind that they find more acceptable.

The ancient Zen teacher Chao-chou said in a dharma talk to his students, "Buddhahood is passion, and passion is Buddhahood." A student asked him, "In whom does Buddha cause passion?" Chao-chou answered, "Buddha causes passion in all of us." The student asked, "How do we get rid of it?" Chao-chou: "Why should we get rid of it?"

For many years, I flatly denied that I felt any anger and struggled with the various forms it took when it was denied, like passive-aggressive behavior, sarcasm, and negativism. As I practiced meditation and my foibles became less threatening to me, I finally came to recognize anger in myself. I mean by that that I came to recognize what it actually felt like to be angry. Then I had the problem of how best to handle this feeling, whether to express or suppress it. But that was a separate issue. Initially, I was just thrilled to finally feel something I could identify as anger. The woman in the following story was my first teacher in this matter: she could *feel* her anger! And further, she wanted to present it to me, her antagonist. I think the sparks that flew between us that day opened up to me the range of possibilities in relationships. We eventually became very close friends.

When I was a new student at Zen Center's Green Gulch Farm, my husband, infant son, and I shared a little house with another similarly compositioned family. Our two-room residences were separated by a tiny shared kitchen and bathroom. Though we were all expected to follow the same monastic schedule at Green Gulch, and we all did so, our two families had opposite habits. Tony and I put our baby to bed early. He was asleep before our 9:00 PM meditation, and we returned from the meditation hall at 9:45 to collapse into our beds and absorb every possible millisecond of sleep before our rising time of 4:30 AM. John and Margaret, on the other hand, were dealing with a colicky baby. Sometimes he would cry late into the night.

Adding to this tension was the fact that we all had different ideas of how dishes should be done, the shower cleaned, and how often such things should happen. There was a lot of tension between the two couples, especially Margaret and me. Both of us exaggerated the steadiness of our voices whenever we discussed who had last done the dishes. Finally, on one particular day, things came to a head. She lit into me, burying me in a barrage of articulate criticism about what was wrong with me, why nobody liked me, how arrogant I was, and so on. She was very specific and had obviously devoted a great deal of thought to my faults. Although I had had my difficulties with coworkers and roommates in the past, nobody had ever confronted me so directly before. I felt helpless. The only way I knew of to hold up my side of this argument was to hurl at her every obscenity I knew of concerning her gender, her mother's sexual habits, and her private parts.

She seemed quite startled by my reaction. Here she was offering her best in terms of constructive criticism, and I was merely obscene. When she mentioned the incident in passing to Reb Anderson, he called me in. "Margaret told me what you said to her," he began. I nodded resentfully, not seeing why I, the injured one, should be called on the carpet like this. "What state of mind do you think you were in when you said those things to her?" I knew he was referring to the Buddhist text that all of us at Green Gulch were studying at the time, the *Abhidharma,* which listed the possible states of mind as "wholesome, unwholesome, and neutral." I thought about it. I hadn't seemed to myself to be especially disturbed during my encounter with Margaret. I was just trying to save face by holding up my end of an argument. "I guess I was in a neutral state of mind," I said. "You think you were in a neutral state of mind?" he repeated, clearly astonished. "You're like a lamb with a machine gun! If you can't even recognize your own anger, how can you protect other people from it?"

I was stunned by this information. Not only at his certainty that I had been angry when all I had felt was numb; the notion that I might ever be able to be angry and deliberately protect other people from my anger was earthshaking to me. Though it would be several years before I understood what he said to me that day, that confrontation with Margaret—the way she had attempted to engage me—and the meeting with him were at least the beginning of my constructive confusion on the topic.

Most immediately, however, failing to understand what he was talking about, I remained in denial about ever having been angry. I didn't even put two and two together—that my characteristic numbness when I was wronged was actually unfelt anger. Also, at that time, the early seventies, there was very little encouragement to investigate anger around Zen Center. On the contrary, it even seemed dangerous to do so. I was glad that I was a represser rather than an expresser because I saw what censure more expressive Zen students brought down upon themselves. Very often I agreed privately with whoever was complaining that injustice was being done when someone was being hurt by some policy or other. But if whoever raised the issue did it in an indignant or cranky way, the presentation itself seemed to become the focus of the discussion. The real issue would get lost as people tsked-tsked over the excessive emotion of the presenter. "Soooo angry," someone would say, implying that the complainer was not thorough enough in her efforts to practice Zen, and that would be the end of that. I wondered how things could ever change if righteous anger is unacceptable? And furthermore, if expressing anger is unacceptable in a Zen community, how can anger be dealt with as a spiritual practice?

It finally came to a personal head for me several years ago in a meeting of my women's group when one woman said to another that she would never tell her anything substantial because she was afraid this woman would get too upset, she had such a low tolerance for any sort of conflict. I was immediately furious on behalf of my friend, the woman to whom this was said. I heatedly told the woman who had spoken to her, "If you had said such a thing to me, I would never speak to you again!" Everyone was shocked into silence, it was such an uncharacteristic outburst of direct anger from me. I never was direct with my anger. I was usually sarcastic or passive-aggressive.

The meeting continued, and we were civil, but I could no longer concentrate on our interaction. What interested me personally about what I'd said—what was about to change my life—was how emotionally brittle I must be to feel the way I had expressed in the meeting. And when I went home and began to examine my emotional past, I found it was true. I had broken off relations with several people over the years, even men I was going to marry, because they had disappointed me in some way. They failed some unconscious test of devotion or did something I felt constituted a betrayal. And when they did that, that was it for me: no discussion, no negotiation, no nothing. I remembered a conversation from years ago in which a boyfriend protested that the reason I gave for not seeing him again—that he didn't call me often enough between dates—must not be the real reason; it was so "lame," he said. He was absolutely right; my reason for not continuing the relationship was that he'd said something about me that conflicted with my own view of myself. Instead of complaining to him about my hurt feelings, I just ended the relationship.

This had happened many times in my life, and after the incident at my women's group meeting, I began to question the way I handled my hurt, my resentment. Despite my age and years of meditation practice, I was clearly as primitive emotionally as a child. Although I seemed to myself to have matured in various ways from the person I was as a young woman—I was more able to consider the complexities in situations, to hold opposing views rather than simplifying problems just to be consistent—in this huge area of handling emotions, I was still very immature. If I was hurt by a friend, I never fully trusted that person again; in essence, I ended the friendship.

Another thing that seemed related to my inability to absorb disappointment in relationship was that when other people appeared to be upset over something I had said or done, I often had no idea what it was they were talking about. Someone would say I must be angry at him or her, because of how I had spoken and what I had said, and what was the problem between us? I would reply, "No, I'm not angry at you; you misinterpreted that." Naturally the person was puzzled, but what could he or she say? I had denied it. Suddenly, because of that night at my women's group meeting, it occurred to me that I must be cut off from a huge part of myself.

I decided to ask myself again and again for as long as it took to get an answer: What would it be like to feel anger? To really feel it completely, starting with the stirrings, and then instead of cutting it off and going numb or jumping into my so-called higher self and explaining it away, thereby "taming" it in the only way I knew, trying instead to just sit there in the middle of it and letting it run its whole course? So I began doing this.

The first thing I noticed was that I didn't have many emotions at all, and when I did have them, they didn't last very long. They immediately changed into some sort of numbness. That numbness got better defined in time, as I observed it closely, and it was actually more like muddleheadedness, woolheadedness, like having a really bad head cold. After a while, I came to understand that this was my substitute for feeling because I was really frightened to feel anything in front of another person, especially if such a feeling would make me the center of attention, like at meetings. If something upset me, I got confused and muddled, unable to think. I saw over time that this was such a reliable indication that I was angry that I started acting on it as if I really felt my anger. I began saying at meetings, "Wait, something is wrong here. I don't know what, but something is off." And this worked very well. People would stop and process my objection, because, of course, I was rarely the only one who felt something awry. But now, with my new determination to ferret out my anger, I was often the first person to say something was wrong.

Another thing I noticed when I started looking for my anger was that, on some preconscious level I hadn't been aware of, I kept track of every little hurt done me by anyone else, and I settled all my scores, every one. I used whatever means I had at my disposal to do nasty little things to people, passive-aggressive things that couldn't be directly protested: I'd never have any money on hand for certain people to cash checks when I was treasurer at Green Gulch Farm; or I would agree to help someone out (he had asked for my help without realizing that he was flying into a spider's web) but then conveniently "forget" to do it; or I might say something really spiteful in a reasoned tone of voice, pretending (and some part of myself really believing) that I was giving honest feedback instead of intentionally hurting someone; or I would be really elusive to someone who needed my cooperation as part of her job.

All this nastiness on my part went on at the same time that I was also consciously kind and generous and energetically helpful.

To this day, I'm frankly amazed that I wasn't murdered by some frustrated person who just couldn't take the craziness anymore. Passive-aggressive behavior is a particularly terrible adjustment to being unable to acknowledge your anger. Not only is it really hard on everyone around you, but you yourself can't figure out why people don't respond to you the way you expect and why they don't treat you as kindly in the same situations in which they extend their goodwill to other people.

When I worked in a kitchen years ago, there was a woman there who was maybe the angriest, most vicious coworker I have ever had. This woman was terrible indeed to work with. She saw herself as a victim, protecting herself against inevitable aggression, but she was completely unaware of how she provoked that aggression from the anguished people around her. She complained relentlessly about the rest of us, her kitchen coworkers, accusing us of avoiding her when she needed our help. She had no hesitation about launching a sudden, seemingly unpremeditated verbal attack on whoever was standing next to her. If the person protested such undeserved treatment, she would deny that she was angry, even in the middle of obvious carnage. She'd put it all on her chosen target, saying, "You're the one who's upset, not me. I'm just trying to work here." It was actually hard not to smack her upside the head, if only to try to cut through all this madness.

I remember one meal prep in which she spent the whole time complaining to the rest of us about her ex-husband, how he used to hit her. We were all completely silent while she told her story of spousal abuse. With great effort, I kept my eyes glued to the counter on which I was working because I didn't dare meet anyone else's eyes, and I knew everyone else was doing the same. Finally when I dared raise my eyes to another coworker, we had to look away again. We were all, to our collective horror, sympathizing with her wife-beating husband! So passive-aggressive behavior is indeed a particularly annoying and ineffective way to handle your anger.

As my practice of staying in my anger continued, the emotion started being more discernible to me. I could recognize the beginning of it and feel it swell, peak, and then fade, running its full course for my observation. So my next question was what to do about my anger. Should I just feel it and know it and not act on it? Or should I express it?

I looked around me for clues. Although it had been a while, I vividly remembered a student at Green Gulch Farm who had been encouraged to express her anger for a time as a practice. It was pretty unpleasant to be around her—for starters, because you never knew when she was going to go off. But I could remember thinking at the time, from watching her explosions alternate with bouts of regret, you could really see what a dead-end strategy unchecked expression was. Her anger never seemed to be alleviated; there didn't seem to be a finite amount that she could use up and get free of. She only ended up feeling bad about what she had said and done to other people during her tantrums, and she was very frustrated that when she was expressing her anger, nobody listened to what she was so upset about. They just tried to get out of the way.

But at least she was directly confronting her demon and using a certain strategy to try to understand it. Many of us less courageous mortals fall into a less revealing trap that I call "jumping to the higher self." This is cutting off feeling right at its beginning rather than trying to work through it and use what it tells us about our fears and yearnings. We rationalize our anger and toss it over our shoulder: "What difference will it make in a hundred years?" "I really should be beyond this by now." "I understand why she did that, so I can forgive her." "He only owes me a few bucks; I shouldn't obsess about his not paying me." This is identifying with an imagined higher, more developed self that has transcended ego. Egolessness is seen as a developmental stage to be attained by rigorous spiritual practice or, in the secular world, by self-discipline. When we do this, we don't give our anger or passions the respect they deserve; they're just temporary irritants we will someday grow beyond.

In this view, meditation (or belief in Jesus) can be used to withdraw from our confusing feelings and distance ourselves from snits over petty annoyances. I think some people even unconsciously enter monastic practice in order to turn away from their problems rather than work them through. As we all know, it's pretty frustrating to try to work out a disagreement with people like this, or even discuss an issue with them, because they're always jumping out of their real feelings—which would inform them of their actual point of view—into some stance of equanimity. You feel as if you're talking to a zombie with a strained smile. "Jumping to the higher self" is a way of not dealing with or expressing anger. As I searched for examples of skillful handling of emotion, I saw this all around me, but I knew it wasn't for me any longer.

If we interpret passages like those I mentioned earlier in the *Abhidharma* about "man's untamed and unbridled emotive nature" as a directive to suppress a part of us we view as undeveloped or inferior to other parts of us, we set up a big problem for ourselves. Character traits we don't like in ourselves and try to suppress are actually made more powerful by attempts to stamp them out. We give them a lot of energy and prominence if we're always paying attention to them, noticing them with considerable impatience, and then trying to cut them off. Not to mention that all the frustration engendered by this great effort is for naught. Herbert Guenther points out in his *Philosophy and Psychology in the Abhidharma,* that the *Abhidharma* itself, the source of that irritating quote about "man's untamed and unbridled emotive nature," declares that "[w]e cannot effectively repress emotions; impulses continue to be active and contribute to the perception of the world in a distorted manner. The disturbances by emotion will be removed only by changes in interpretation. With insight and wisdom, the tranquil equanimity of Nirvana is attained by a radical change of attitude." Now here we have something: "a radical change of attitude."

UNCURBED IN ETERNAL GLORY

What seemed after a while to be most satisfying for me in dealing with my anger was holding the feeling without judging it, feeling it in my body, staying in it for as long as it lasted, then watching it change of its own accord into something else. I found after doing this for some time that real spaciousness developed around the angry thoughts and feelings themselves. When I was able to recognize my feelings and hold them close and feel the space around them, I felt as if I had a choice about openly expressing them. So for me, this was indeed a "radical change in attitude," since my original problem was not that I was expressing explosively but that I was expressing indirectly.

I began to be able to use the energy my anger stirred in me for my own needs, to fuel action or to pay attention to some difficulty I might have dismissed as too petty, not important enough to follow up on. Finally, as Reb had intimated was possible in that long-ago discussion at Green Gulch Farm, I began to be able to protect people from my anger. What incredible power that seemed to be! I could be angry, could feel hurt and undermined, and express it to whoever I felt had hurt me, in a way that allowed space for the person to stay in the situation and listen to me, just by including space for the other's point of view when I approached him or her. "Maybe you didn't mean that the way I took it because it really hurt me, and I'm pretty angry about it now. I want to talk with you about it and find out what you were thinking."

Suddenly I was wholly relational! Not just having relationships in good times, in the sunshine, but also in the bad times, during the stormy struggles. I can't tell you how that opened my world! I began to understand that if you pay enough attention to develop skill at it—using the energy from your anger to inspire you to express yourself, but not aiming it at anyone else—anger can actually make a situation between people suddenly intimate because it gives you the impetus to cut through social distance.

As the years have passed, my anger has become a welcome friend to me. In the process, I have come to understand that neither suppression nor explosive expression nor even peaceful expression is my only option in dealing with anger. We can hold feelings in the "balance of meditative equipoise," as Mark Epstein calls it in *Thoughts without a Thinker,* "so that they can be seen in a clear light." When I began to try to be aware of my anger, I had to start at the beginning, with the mind that got woolheaded when I was hurt and childishly kept track of other people's slights. Only by paying precise attention to those states of mind every time I was quick enough to notice them, trying to discern exactly what I was experiencing, moment after moment, could I finally locate my true feeling, hidden beneath layers of protection. This is not a fun practice. You really squirm when you see yourself this way: hurt over the most ridiculous things, driven nearly to tears by other people's most inconsequential behaviors, which you may even have misinterpreted in the first place. But as Epstein points out, "it is the fundamental tenet of Buddhism that this kind of attention is in itself healing."

As space around it opened up for me, I began to realize how complex anger is. It's not just one thing; it's multilayered and intricate. In some of its forms, it's destructive to both the person expressing it and the person on the receiving end; this is violence. But in some other forms, it is extremely useful. When I was first crippled with arthritis, I often had wild, thrashing, sobbing temper tantrums that expressed my loss and grief at going from a competent young woman to a hobbled dependent. But as time passed and I sank into my life as just my life rather than as a living hell, my level of mundane suffering decreased enormously. So I expected my frequent short bursts of rage—my temper tantrums—to subside. After all, I was experiencing less rage and frustration, although my life was certainly still full of struggles with bedsheets and jar lids. At that time, I thought of my temper tantrums as indications of some basic inability to cope with my pain, so naturally I expected them to go away eventually.

My current view is absolutely the opposite. I've come to think over the years that opting to have a temper tantrum is one of the healthiest things I do. Short bursts of rage can be extremely restorative if we live with the constant frustration of chronic pain or extreme stress. We must give vent to these feelings as often as we feel comfortable doing so. It's very hard to value these feelings because we've been taught so consistently as children that we must never lose control in such an extreme way, but I say if we take certain precautions—that there is never any danger of hurting ourselves or anyone else—let 'er rip!

A woman said to me recently that she admired how accepting I am of my pain, that she, also in a lot of pain, could never be so accepting as I appear to be. She said dolefully, obviously yearning for my great wisdom, that instead of being serene like me, she's always angry at her pain. I laughed, recalling my oft-rendered shrieks and curses—and envisioning the woman's probable reaction if she could interview my family and discover my real behavior—and said to her that I thought a big part of "accepting your pain" (her words) is knowing for sure that you are entitled to be angry as hell! And that it seems really healthy and rejuvenating to find as many ways as you can to express that bitterness.

For instance, my family is familiar with my everyday frustration with household objects that my arthritic hands can no longer manipulate effectively. More than one morning, I have been unable to loosen the lid on the jam jar to put jam on my warm, newly buttered toast. I try and try with all my might—the toast is lying there on the napkin, drooling with butter, exuding tasty aroma—and if I can just get this lid off, I can have my toast and jam immediately.

But I can't. I twist and twist, run the jar hastily under the hot water, wrap a towel around it, try a can opener made especially for arthritic hands (it never works for me, though when I'm desperate, I try it yet again, thinking this time it *will* work), but this morning nothing will budge the jam jar lid. Yesterday I could open it, but this morning either someone else has tightened it too tight, the sugar has hardened around the lid, or my fingers are weaker than yesterday.

On this particular day, it just came down to too many frustrating bouts with inanimate objects that I always lose. Overcome with the ineffectualness of my adult body, convinced I was the only person in America not having jam with my toast, I suddenly hurled the jam jar against the kitchen wall. It crashed there, and the jam started slowly oozing down the wall toward the floor, cluttered with broken glass shards. I admit it—I was shocked at myself. But that surprise was immediately replaced with a tremendously warm and satisfied feeling, which spread across my chest and belly. I may not have had jam, but I did have my revenge. It was sweet, as sweet as any jam, and glorious. I ate my buttered toast with great pleasure as I watched the jam make its slow but inexorable journey to the linoleum floor. It just so happened that that morning the radio was blaring the alarming news that some maniac had just shot his ex-wife and was running from justice. As I sat there crunching on my toast, listening to the report, I thought darkly, "I know why he did that. He couldn't get the lid off the *@#*! jam jar!"

Maybe I hadn't been able to conquer, but at least I could destroy. I was so pleased with the feeling of triumph it caused, I left the jam there on the wall and floor until evening. Every time I entered the kitchen I viewed it with pleasure. I refused to let my husband or son take care of it since I wanted to continue to feel my own power. I cleaned it up just before I went to bed that night. Since that day, I have repeated that deeply satisfying violent gesture a couple of times. The last time, my son came into the kitchen, saw the splattered mess, and sighed, "Oh, Mom, not another jam jar." We took to buying our jam in quantity.

Now, years later, I have become quite skilled at having temper tantrums. Since I immediately start paying attention to angry feelings when they first begin to rise, I have time to make a choice about whether to hold them and run through their course on my own or to indulge them and involve other people. It is in this spirit that I decided some time ago to begin to allow myself to have temper tantrums in certain public situations. I have found them invaluable for cutting through the bureaucratese and job resentment that often make service people so impervious to the customers they are paid to assist. By stating my anger clearly without directing it at any specific person who would then need to defend himself or herself, I've been able to forge communication with people who were impenetrable at first: indifferent clerks, vainglorious telephone company supervisors, arrogant doctors, stressed-out health care providers, smug mechanics, and even Zen practitioners.

Here's an example from my own life:

ME (*having reached the service department of a large mail-order company after days of getting a busy signal*): Hi, I'm calling you about a problem.

SERVICE REPRESENTATIVE: What is your problem?

ME: I ordered a nightstand from you last month, and it was missing the front door. When I called to ask you to send me the door, you sent me another nightstand, which is also missing the front door. I only want one nightstand, but I want it with a front door. Would you send me a front door, and would you have UPS come and pick up the extra nightstand?

SERVICE REPRESENTATIVE: I'm sorry, but we can't pay for UPS to pick it up. You'll have to take it to a post office and mail it to us.

ME (*annoyed, becoming aware of the possibility that this conversation might not end in my customer satisfaction*): Well, that seems a little unreasonable, considering that it is your fault I have two nightstands and no front door.

SERVICE REPRESENTATIVE: I'm sorry, but that's our policy.

ME: Let me get this straight. Even though it was due to your company's error that I got an extra nightstand, you are asking me to find some way of getting this piece of furniture to a post office and then paying to return it?

SERVICE REPRESENTATIVE: We will, of course, pay for the postage. We just can't pay for anyone to pick it up.

ME (*beginning to understand from my rising anger that a decision about whether to have a tantrum is imminent*): I can't get this to a post office! I have trouble walking!

SERVICE REPRESENTATIVE: Maybe you could get a friend to do it.

ME (*I decide to go for it but do not wish to demolish the service representative, impervious though she seems. I attempt to protect her despite my genuine anger.*): Listen, I understand that this is not your company and that you don't make policy. But your refusal to take any responsibility for your company's error is driving me crazy! (*My voice rises, and I get more emotional as I go.*) I called asking for help in solving a problem your company caused, and you present more problems! I demand that you pick up this *@#*! extra nightstand and send me a *@#*! front door for the other one!!

SERVICE REPRESENTATIVE (*shaken at last*): I'll get my supervisor to speak to you, ma'am.

ME (*genuinely*): Thank you!

SUPERVISOR: Can I help you, Ms. Cohen?

ME (*still upset but enjoying the catharsis*): Yes, thank God you're on the phone! I'm really upset that your company sent me two nightstands when I only ordered one—neither one has a front door—and you won't do me the courtesy of picking up one of them. You want me to somehow lug it to a post office and mail it to you!

SUPERVISOR (*guarded, but not distracted*): Yes, that's our policy, Ms. Cohen. If you want to send it UPS, you would have to pay the extra charge for picking it up.

ME (*really furious now, the thrill of release surging through my veins*): What? That's *@#*! outrageous! I'll tell you what I'm going to do: I'm going to call UPS, have them pick up *both* nightstands, and refuse to pay UPS or you for either one! You can take me to court for it! I want to tell you, I don't usually carry on like a madwoman, but you have driven me to it by your refusal to deal fairly with the problems you caused me!!

SUPERVISOR (*obviously dealing with a crazy person, so becomes soothing*): I can understand your frustration, Ms. Cohen, and we want to solve this.

ME (*exploding*): Then *@#*! do what I *@#*! ask! Do you know what it's like to get the nightstand you've been waiting for, and it doesn't have any front door?! Then you call up the company to send you a front door, and they send you another nightstand, and now you have two useless nightstands blocking the hallway, and they refuse to pick up one of them and send you a front door for the other one?!

SUPERVISOR (*suddenly very, very calm*): All right, Ms. Cohen, we will pick up the second nightstand, since it was our error.

ME (*somewhat taken aback*): You will? You really will?

SUPERVISOR: Yes, just repack it for us, and put this identification number on the label on the front of the package. We will reimburse you.

ME: Will you reimburse me for this long phone call as well?

SUPERVISOR: Yes.

ME: And will you send me a front door?

SUPERVISOR (*genuinely conciliatory*): Of course.

ME (*feeling moved by her kindness*): I want to thank you so much for taking care of me this way. I'm sorry I was so upset, but you understand.

SUPERVISOR: OK, Ms. Cohen. Will $5 cover the phone call?

ME: I think so.

SUPERVISOR: I'll send you a separate check for the phone call and deduct the UPS cost from your credit card charge.

ME: Thank you so much.

SUPERVISOR: Have a good day.

My point in recounting this long, tiresome exchange is not that I got what I wanted, though that certainly was important to me at the time, but rather that I was able to weave my strong feeling into the exchange in such a way that it forged a connection in a way that being polite could not. The supervisor was sincere when she wished me a good day at the end. We had met each other. At that point, it sounded to me as if she actually felt good about having been able to take care of me. She did not sound as if she had lost a battle. On the contrary, she had succeeded in handling a very difficult customer with consideration and goodwill. We both won.

Thich Nhat Hanh deserves the last word: "Treat your anger with the utmost respect and tenderness, for it is no other than yourself. Do not suppress it—simply be aware of it. Awareness is like the sun. When it shines on things, they are transformed. When you are aware that you are angry, your anger is transformed. If you destroy anger, you destroy the Buddha, for Buddha and Mara are of the same essence. Mindfully dealing with anger is like taking the hand of a little brother."

PART THREE

HOW TO BE ALIVE FOR EVERYTHING

8

ACCESSING THE BODY'S WISDOM

❧

ALWAYS BUSY

WE Americans are a nation of compulsive workers who prefer activity with end products, like contracts or new cars, to activity that has no visible goal, like meditation or sitting in the sun. We admire and emulate people who are very good at producing a great deal of evidence of their efforts—such as corporation presidents, sports figures, or movie producers. Since we evaluate people based on what they produce and consume, we all wish to prove our worth by showing how much we can do. We fill our days with tasks and have five- and ten-year plans for our entire lives. We always have a feeling of racing against time. We wear watches on our wrists and constantly check them to see how we're doing.

When we go on vacation, we have an opportunity to escape the pressure to produce and the feeling of being trapped by time, but for many of us, productivity is such a powerful habit that we continue to pile up the achievements, merely substituting play activities for work tasks rather than living differently altogether: so many laps in the pool, getting up early in order to finish a round of golf by lunch in order to squeeze in a tour before dinner. If we can't even relax when no specific demands are being made on us, it's no wonder so many of us lead hectic, stress-filled lives completely estranged from the feelings in our own bodies.

Even when we intentionally turn our attention to our bodies, as when we do physical exercise, we tend to maintain our goal orientation. We devise an exercise *program* rather than directly feeling our bodies' yearnings. We work out in order to become stronger and healthier rather than for any pleasure afforded us by the actual doing of the activity. In fact, statistics showing that most of us soon abandon our workout programs make it clear that we get no pleasure from these physical exercise routines.

When you lead a goal-oriented life, you pay attention to your ideas, your plans, and your expectations rather than to your feelings and the sensations of your body. Your body becomes little more than the mobile equipment that gets you across the street and to your appointments. In your daily life, you focus on your ideas about your abilities and what you ought to accomplish. Your body intrudes on your goal-oriented consciousness only to demand food or sleep and to register pain. In this situation, your body never gets a chance to relax, to be itself, to please itself; it is always at the disposal of your head-derived concepts and goals. You may continue your relentless push to achieve, to accomplish, until you develop some serious physical or emotional difficulty that interferes with your functioning.

Many of us are so preoccupied with thoughts and worries that we hardly register any sensations at all. Let's say we decide to go to the bank. It's a few blocks away, and because of the parking problem, it's easier to walk. We start off down the street. Maybe we are thinking of what will happen when we get to the bank. Will we have enough in the account to cover our withdrawal? What if we get that annoying teller? What if we have to stand in line? What are we planning to do after leaving the bank? What else might be the focus of our minds as we walk along? The sweet spring air as it brushes our cheek? The sensation of our feet hitting the pavement, causing vibration in our feet and knees? The sensation of our clothes against our skin as our muscles move? The sounds of traffic in our ears? These are all internal, timeless, sensate experiences of moving through space. No goal is connected with any of them; our brains are simply organizing the information they receive through our five senses. For some of us, the details of the past or future occupy the mind to the exclusion of any of the actual sensations we might feel while walking to the bank. Unfortunately, the ability to register the sensations of the body may atrophy as a muscle does if it is never used.

We may think ahead, make plans, establish goals, but we don't have to do that every moment. Actually, we don't need to think about the end results of our activity very often at all. We decide to complete a project, and we begin the work. We might have to check the time or the calendar periodically to see that we are progressing well enough to meet any deadline, but otherwise, we are free to actually live through our experience of completing the tasks. We can live through the activity—typing a term paper, creating a book proposal, folding the laundry, preparing a meal—feeling our muscle movements, aware of our various thoughts and feelings, sensing the movement of our clothes across our bodies. Noting our compulsion to worry about the next activity as just that, a compulsion, we can move on to the next thought or sensation.

Doing a job from the viewpoint of our bodies requires that we develop the mental flexibility to shift back and forth between our ideational, decision-making mind and the physical sensations of our bodies. All the actual movements we make—reaching for the phone, settling in our chairs—can be done with our minds focused on our bodily feelings. Planning, creating, and problem solving require focusing on abstract concepts, but even so, we can drop in periodically to check out bodily sensations.

Why should we develop the ability to feel sensations? Aside from the philosophical questions of the richness of life and the emotional satisfaction to be had from experiencing events on many different levels, if we do develop some physical difficulty or our lives are interrupted by pain, sensation is where we need to go to find out how to alleviate pain. I must emphasize that there is nothing wrong with using the intellect, nor is there anything inferior about our brains compared to our bodies. We plan in order to have the resources to enjoy our lives. We make appointments so that we can conduct business and share pleasure with each other. We must be careful, however, not to get stuck in any one aspect of our rich and multidimensional selves. We benefit enormously from experiences of our unbounded, timeless natures as well as our smart, linear brains; access to the timeless kinds of experiences lies in our feelings and sensations.

As Bernie Siegel points out in his fascinating book *Love, Medicine and Miracles,* we have no agreed-upon way in our culture to withdraw for a while and get more familiar with a deeper part of ourselves that is not interested in the preoccupations of our ordinary lives: making enough money, getting dinner on the table, winning the approval of our friends and acquaintances. In many other cultures, it is commonplace to retreat from everyday life for a prescribed time and get in touch with the aspect of ourselves that is not goal-directed and time-oriented, that is not concerned with gaining or losing, but is boundless and infinite. I call this aspect The One Who Is Not Busy.

Encountering the One Who Is Not Busy

To come into contact with The One Who Is Not Busy, we soften the specific focus that we usually bring to our daily concerns and start paying attention not just to what furthers our goals but to everything inside us and around us. Our perspective on life radically changes when we have no concerns but being aware. We get a chance to see how information comes in through our senses and evokes thoughts and feelings. Our daily preoccupations drop away, and we come to know what basic awareness is like, before we put layers and layers of concerns on top of it. If we pay close attention, we can see quite clearly the process by which we pile on those layers of concerns. Getting back to basic awareness is like peeling an onion until we reach the core, ground zero for our thoughts and feelings.

If we are to live comfortably with pain and drastically reduce the stress it causes us, we must quiet the voices that are always clamoring for our attention: the voice of goal direction (what we must accomplish), the voices of our fantasies (what it would be like if we won the lottery or were universally recognized as a wonderful person), the voice of compulsion (what tasks we need to be doing instead of what we're actually doing at this moment), and the voice of reassurance (endlessly shoring up our sense of self and security). If these voices are quieted a little from time to time, other realities may have a chance to come forward and be noticed: the sounds of our organs working, our breathing, the animal presence of other beings who are in the same room with us, and sounds that are usually in the background of our main focus, like children playing or cars passing. We might be able to notice that our thoughts have some compulsive pattern that is repeated over and over again. When we notice patterns like that, we have a *choice* about whether to continue to follow a particular pattern rather than helplessly following it whenever it pops up in our minds.

In other words, when we are consciously aware of our bodies and the whole sensual environment around us, we create for ourselves an opportunity to notice what's usually overwhelmed by our daily preoccupations. If we can get in touch with the sensations of our bodies, sitting still or moving, we may suddenly feel all the profoundly nourishing connections that our ordinary life does not include, like the fact that we sit on this planet earth, that our breath goes in and out continuously, that our bones shift when we change our posture. This is encountering The One Who Is Not Busy.

The most creative people among us are those who are able to break the grip of habit-based thinking and take some other point of view from time to time. Gary Larson makes us laugh by taking animals' points of view in his cartoons; a good lawyer can switch back and forth from the defendant's to the prosecutor's point of view to test his client's case; a photographer finds the most dramatic or aesthetically pleasing point of view from which to record an event; an investor looks at business from the point of view of increasing her funds. For people who want to improve the function of their bodies, it is most advantageous to see things from the body's point of view. The realm of The One Who Is Not Busy is also the domicile of the timeless, boundless healer.

If much of our lives is lived from the viewpoint of our bodies, we begin to heal ourselves from stress and pain every waking moment. If we take our bodies' point of view and begin to receive and understand their messages, our bodies will tell us how to take care of them. Most of us already have some familiarity with living this way. If we go on vacation, we have an opportunity to "eat when we want to eat" instead of at prescribed, conventional times and "sleep when we want to sleep" instead of all at once at a certain time. We exert ourselves when we feel energetic and relax when we feel lethargic.

Most of us cannot do this in our daily lives because our schedules do not allow eating when we are hungry, napping when we are tired, running or playing tennis when we feel high-spirited, lounging when we feel like "not doing much of anything." We do know, however, what it feels like to live that way because most of us have lived that way when we are home from work with a cold; then we do whatever we feel like doing—it's like a time-out from our usual lives. A great advantage of taking our bodies' point of view while we move about is that we can begin to use the routines and tasks of our own daily lives to restore our well-being. We can reverse a physical difficulty or heighten vibrant good health and enrich our lives so that they are much more satisfying by getting familiar with doing things from our bodies' point of view.

How can you begin to live in the world from the point of view of your body? Begin with feeling your body now as you read this. What are you doing, actually? Feel your eyes moving as you follow the printed words on the page. Feel the weight of the book in your hand or on your lap. Feel how your spine supports your neck, your back. Feel the tension level in your legs. Are they relaxed where they are? Do they yearn to stretch, move, flex? Feel your jaw, your neck, your shoulders. Become aware of any feelings that make one part of your body stand out in your consciousness from other parts. You may feel pain and tension. Try adjusting your posture to ease tension if you can. You may feel nothing at all that draws your attention. In that case, move your hand, then your arm, and feel what changes the movements produce in those parts and in the areas around those parts. Begin to get familiar with what it feels like to move, to prepare to move, to change the body's position. Become aware of muscle tension that yearns to be relieved by moving.

Movement is what muscles like to do. That is their preoccupation, their goal in life. Our muscles are connected by nerve cells to our brains. We have a feedback system in which our brains not only tell our muscles what to do (take us to the bank, chop vegetables for dinner) but orchestrate the release of tension. We all yawn and stretch to accommodate the messages of our muscles. We can get very sensitive to these messages. We can shift them into the center of our consciousness instead of leaving them at the periphery. During the course of our daily lives, we move anyway. We might as well learn to move so that our movements increase our well-being rather than strain, constrict, and exhaust our bodies.

Why would we, in our ordinary lives, want to check in again and again with our bodies? It might be annoying to do so while we're immersed in a great run on the computer. Computer work is compulsively cerebral: one thought leads to another, which leads to another, which leads to another, and so on. It takes tremendous intention to interrupt this cerebral flow in order to do anything else. Why bother? For starters, we might want to develop more of ourselves as persons than one dimension. We might want to experience something in our lives besides our thinking, decision-making brain. We all have aspects of the poet, the artist, the scientist, the lover. What a shame to be only a one-trick pony in our lives! Awareness of a bodily sensation or a sense impression dramatically broadens our scope, our reality. It gives us some perspective on our discursive minds; it shows us that they're not the only—or even the sanest—game in town.

It's inherently sane, real, to be connected with and aware of the physical and sensual aspects of our activity as well as its purpose. It is an expression of sanity to be so intimately connected to our activity that we can allow a broom to sweep us just as we sweep the broom, that we can appreciate this relationship we are having with the broom. By giving our daily movements our full attention, our minds have a chance to unfold, revealing psychic space around pain, space around frustration, space around everything. This kind of space is always there in our psyches, available to receive us. The One Who Is Not Busy is always there, aware of our muscles working, aware of the breeze on our cheeks. We develop the ability to turn at will to The One Who Is Not Busy by noticing very simple experiences: the sudden whiff of fresh air when we step outside onto the porch; the sudden dimming and narrowing of space when we step inside a building; the warmth of a mug of tea cupped in our palms; the instant of palpable satisfaction from placing a heavy cup on the table—when we perceive the precise meeting of two flat surfaces. These are real experiences of being alive; we usually ignore them as mundane, but they are the ways we can know The One Who Is Not Busy.

When we are connected to The One Who Is Not Busy, our activity itself expresses our deepest unobstructed nature. When we live to express this unfettered nature, we are intimately connected to our desires, our thoughts and feelings, our bodies. We take care of our bodies because they yearn to be taken care of and we feel generous toward them. We are aware when we want to rest, to eat, when we need stimulation, when we want to challenge ourselves. We are sometimes indulgent and sometimes firm with our bodies, as with a child. If our bodies disappoint us, as when we have lost functioning that we once had, or we feel impatient with our bodies because they no longer obey our commands like slaves, we can practice letting them have their way or gently directing them here or there. We can tell them firmly that they must prepare our dinner or take their daily constitutional, but that beyond that, we will indulge them: give them a posture they enjoy, a chance to relax, promising to bathe them in appreciation for what they can do.

Some years ago, an elderly, but still very active, Japanese tea teacher came to me with complaints of pain and swelling in her knees. Not only do tea teachers sit on their knees for the better part of the day, this woman also lived on the third floor of a large building. She was understandably concerned about the function and comfort of her knees. I showed her how to gently massage her knees and dissolve the arthritic swelling by coaxing it into the bloodstream with her fingers. I told her to come back the following week so that I could check on her progress.

When she returned, I asked her to demonstrate the massage technique I had showed her to make certain she was doing it right. She put her fingers on her knees, began massaging gently, then added in a tender voice, "Oh, little knees, all these seventy-three years you have helped me so much, supporting me when I walked, holding me when I taught tea, carrying me up all the stairs in my life. Now, little knees, *I* will take care of *you!*" I was stunned with admiration. Would that all my clients demonstrated such an attitude toward their ailing parts! They would be healed in a week, and I would have nothing to do but hang out with The One Who Is Not Busy!

LEARNING TO TAKE THE BODY'S POINT OF VIEW

Because we are more accustomed in our daily lives to the process of cogitating (planning, reasoning, judging, creating) than to the experience of feeling our bodily sensations and impartially processing our sensory input, most of us need some practice receiving the information our bodies are always sending us. It's strange that we don't automatically know how to dip into our bodies' wisdom. Why do we have to learn something that should be instinctual? The answer is that it is indeed deeply instinctual, but most of us in our postmodern technological world have lost our primal connection to our physical being.

Using Breath to Feel Your Body

Consciousness of your breath is a good way to begin to experience sensation and movement in your body. Most people spend much of their lives unaware of how their breath affects their movements. As long as they *can* move, they take their breath for granted. The breath has tremendous potential for unlocking a restricted body.

If you can feel where in your body your breath expands you when you breathe in and shrinks you when you breathe out, and where it does not expand and shrink you, you can use this awareness to differentiate one part of your body from another. For example, put your hands on your ribs, right under your chest. You will feel them expand and shrink as you breathe in and out. Move your hands to the edges of this movement, where your breath stops moving your body as you breathe in and out. Perhaps that is your chest. You can feel your ribs being differentiated from your chest every time you breathe. You can feel internally that your ribs are one part of you and your chest is another. Breathe more deeply and perhaps you can feel your chest muscles expand when you breathe in, just like your ribs. Perhaps now you can distinguish your whole moving midsection from another part that isn't moving with your breath—for instance, your shoulders. Breathe and feel how your midsection differs from your shoulders. You may think, Of course my midsection differs from my shoulders! How obvious! But *feel* the difference. If you are not used to feeling your body and the differences between its various parts, you may be surprised at how subtle these feelings are, how they have to be repeated several times before they attain clarity. You may be surprised, too, at how intense these feelings are, how they could take up your whole world if you weren't preoccupied instead with the ideas and fantasies that usually hold your attention.

The following breathing exercise will accentuate the separations among parts of your torso that you began to notice in the meditation above. People tell me what an enlivening exercise it is, bringing the whole breathing apparatus of the body into awareness. Begin on a mat on the floor. Use whatever pillows you need under your head or other parts of your body in order to be comfortable.

Wave Breathing

1. Lie on your back. Allow your arms to find a comfortable position. Either stretch your legs out on the floor or bend your knees over a pillow for comfort. Breathe normally for

several breaths, allowing your breath to deepen naturally
as you relax.

2. When you feel relaxed, still breathing in and out in your
   normal way, begin to suck in your stomach with your stomach muscles and puff out your chest with your chest muscles at the same time. Continue to breathe in and out
   through your nose.

3. Then collapse your chest and push out your stomach—just
   the opposite of what you did before.

4. Suck in your stomach and puff out your chest again. The
   sucking and puffing should be gentle movements, not
   abrupt or straining but fluid and slow, with as much control
   as you can manage.

5. Then collapse your chest and push out your stomach, suck
   in your stomach and puff out your chest over and over
   again, creating a wave motion as you go back and forth
   between your chest and your stomach. Your breath continues independently as you use your stomach and chest muscles to alternately puff out and pull in your stomach and
   chest. Now relax and feel what you've done.

Your unrestricted breathing creates a natural rhythm for your
body's movements. If you focus on your breath as you move, your
movements naturally follow that rhythm, and your sense of coordination increases. Stiff, contracted people desperately need the
sense of grace and coordination that breath can lend to movement. People in pain yearn for the spaciousness that breath creates around everything: body parts, movements, thoughts, and
events. If you focus on your breath for even a few minutes, you'll
glimpse an alternate reality that is compelling in its potential to
transform the way you currently endure your pain.

Using Awareness Exercises to Feel Your Body

If we are new to the skill of feeling the sensations of our body as
we move, most of us need to do specific movements that increase
our ability to feel the motion of our body in our everyday activi-

ties. The best kind of awareness exercises are those that involve gentle movements, slowly done, so that the brain can easily track the movement we do, and we can therefore feel the sensations that arise in our muscles and joints.

I have developed a system of small, gentle movements that are easy to do and can be done in all positions—lying, sitting, and standing. These movements require a great deal of consciousness, and therein lies much of their effectiveness. I call them Meditation on Movement. I'm quite fond of these movements. Not only are they pleasant and comforting, they're like traditional sitting meditation, only inside out. In sitting meditation, because you are still, you can observe what is moving: your thoughts, sounds, sense impressions, the world going on outside your windows. When you are moving slowly, and you give your movements that same attention, you will not only notice the sensations in your body produced by the movement, you will also notice what is still. Parts of your body seem to be moving around a focal center profoundly at rest.

Meditation on Movement is a gateway to the home of The One Who Is Not Busy. While you are attending to your precise bodily sensations, which are the focus of these movements, you begin to experience the tension between thought and sensation. In order to feel the intricacies of your movement, you must stop thinking long enough to feel sensation. When you follow a train of thought, you have to ignore your sensations and put your body on automatic pilot. You must do one or the other. This is how movement can soothe muscles contracted with tension and calm a mind frantic with stress. You drop past the tension and stress into the sensation of movement.

Body Awareness Movements. The following movements are intended to be Meditations on Movement—that is, they are done to emphasize sensation and the awareness of the body's moving parts. They require a great deal of attention to breath as well as to the movement of muscles and the isolation of one part of the body from another, and therefore, they tend to interrupt the mind's usual flow of thought patterns. All of them involve laying movement on breath—that is, your primary focus during the movements is the in and out of your breath, and your secondary focus is the movement I am describing. The way you move will tend to follow the rhythm laid down by the way you breathe. Many of these movements are intended to bring physical and psychological comfort. They are rhythmic, with great awareness of breath, and they have the feeling tone of a baby being rocked. The movements also promote body awareness—that is, they are done slowly and precisely enough that your attention can stay on your sensations and your feelings as they are evoked by the small movements that you do. The sequence of movements helps you notice very small differences in the feelings of adjacent muscle groups. Doing these movements, you are thoroughly engaged with bodily sensation, which is a strong antidote to discursive thought.

Thoughts and emotions may arise as well as sensations. It will be helpful to you to notice what kinds of thoughts continually arise during your movements and what kinds of feelings come up when you move certain areas of your body. When you find yourself distracted by thought patterns or emotional reactions to certain of the movements, note your reactions and then gently guide your attention back to the sensations of your body. Be patient and gentle with your attention. It may leave your body sensations over and over again. No matter how many times your attention returns to thoughts, just gently guide it back to your body.

I suggest that you experiment with the amount of time you spend doing each movement. Start with five to seven minutes to try a movement out, to test its potential as a healing exercise for your body. Later you may find that twenty or thirty minutes of your favorite movements really makes a difference in how you feel. Rather than watching a clock if your exercise time is limited, you may find it more relaxing to set a timer, thus allowing yourself to sink into the sensations of your body and leave the constraints of the clock for a while.

Do the movements with as little effort as possible so as to maximize the ease and comfort of your body as well as the healing potential of the movements. The movements on these pages are just suggestions for ways that you might move your body. If you are inclined to change an exercise so that the movement is more pleasant for you to do, please trust that inclination. Your body understands better than any book what movements ease it.

Arm Twist

1. Sit comfortably on a chair and let your arms hang loosely at your sides, with the palms of your hands facing in toward your body.
2. Very slowly, with your thumbs leading the motion, turn your palms out away from your body. Your arms will follow the twisting motion of your wrists. Let your arms, hands, and wrists relax completely; only your thumbs are actively moving, causing your arms, hands, and wrists to turn. Notice the feeling of the turning motion in the muscles of your arm.
3. Turn your palms in toward your body and then out away from your body again. Do this over and over. Notice the difference between your hands when they are facing in toward your body and when they are turned out toward the room. Is the temperature different? Do your muscles feel different?
4. Now relax and feel what the movement has done.

Big Toe Turn

1. Sit on a chair and place your arms in a comfortable position. Make sure your feet reach the floor. If they don't, place a pillow on the floor under them so that they rest on a surface. Breathe deeply, aware of your diaphragm rising and falling.
2. Wiggle your toes and become aware of your feet.
3. Turn your big toes toward each other without actually lifting your feet. Stretch your big toes toward each other and feel how the rest of the foot is pulled along.
4. Release your feet and let the big toes fall away from each other.

5. Repeat again and again. As you slowly move your big toes toward each other and then release your feet so that they fall away, notice the movement this causes in your knees and hips. Your knees and hips are passively moved while your feet cause them to turn in the joint.
6. Now relax and feel what the movement has done.

Shoulder Blade Sway in Chair

1. Sit in a chair facing the back of the chair with legs straddling each side of the chair and hands holding either side of the chair back.
2. Begin to move your upper body from one side to the other, leading with your shoulder blades. As you sway from one side to the other, feel your shoulder blades shift in your upper back. Allow your sides to stretch slightly with this movement. Do it gently enough so that what you feel in your lower back is a slight stretch as you shift your weight, not pain from abrupt movement.
3. Now relax and feel what the movement has done.

Elbow Stretch

1. Sit comfortably in a chair, far enough forward so that your feet rest firmly on the floor in front of you.
2. Attempt to touch your elbows together behind your back by stretching your shoulders back and stretching your arms toward each other behind you. It doesn't matter if your elbows can't actually touch; just the effort of bringing them together will stretch the muscles of your upper body.
3. Then bring your arms forward. Let them hang straight between your knees. Attempt to touch your elbows together in front by twisting your arms toward each other until your elbows meet. As you twist your arms, the backs of the hands will come together as well. It doesn't matter if your elbows can't actually touch; just the effort of stretching them toward each other will stretch the muscles of your upper back.

4. Attempt to bring your elbows together behind your back again. Then again in front. Breathe normally, allowing your breath to go in and go out at its own pace as you move. Continue to touch your elbows together in back and in front until you feel stretched in your upper back and chest.
5. When you have become accustomed to moving your arms forward and then back, synchronize your head movements with your arm movements: let your head fall gently forward when you stretch your elbows toward each other in front and let your head fall gently back when you stretch your elbows toward each other behind your back.
6. Relax and feel how the movement has affected the feeling of your upper body and arms.

Breastbone Flex

1. Sit comfortably on a chair with your hands on your knees. Breathe normally, allowing your breath to go in and out without effort.
2. Put your fingers on your breastbone, the large, prominent bone between your breasts. Breathe in and feel the breastbone rise against your fingers. Breathe out and feel it recede from your fingers.
3. Begin to accentuate the rising-and-falling motion by adding the power of your chest muscles to the motion of your breathing. Push your breastbone out when you breathe in and collapse your breastbone between your shoulders when you breathe out. Move just your breastbone alone, not your shoulders or back. This is a very subtle motion for most of us, but it profoundly affects the tension most of us carry in our upper backs. If you succeed in moving your breastbone but cannot do it without moving your shoulders or upper back as well, continue trying to isolate your breastbone movement from the movement of your shoulders, back, or ribs until at last you have the small but powerful rise and fall of your breastbone alone.
4. Relax and feel the sensations that the movement has caused in your chest and back.

Knees Together and Apart

1. Sit on the edge of a chair so that your feet are firmly on the ground, your knees together.
2. Lift your feet, move your legs apart to the edges of the chair, touch the ground briefly, and then move your legs back together again. Do this movement rapidly and lightly, loosening up your hips and thighs. Let your feet lead the motion, allowing your hips to relax and follow along. Don't drag your feet with your hips.
3. Stop and feel what the movement has done.

Raise and Lower Bent Legs

1. Sit on the edge of a chair so that your feet are firmly on the ground with a little distance between them.
2. Lift your right leg (knee bent) off the ground, continuing as high as your leg will comfortably go, then allow it to slowly sink back down to the ground. Do this motion with your foot as the leader: your foot pushes your leg up and pulls it back down to the ground. This avoids the feeling of your hip straining to lift your leg.
3. Repeat with your left foot and leg.
4. Continue to alternate your left and right feet, raising and lowering your bent legs.
5. Stop and feel the feeling the movement has produced in your legs and hips.

Pelvic Rock in Chair

1. Sit in a chair with your feet on the ground. It is not necessary to sit away from the back of the chair. You can rest your spine on the back of the chair.
2. Put your hand on your lower spine just above your buttocks. These are the vertebrae you want to move in this exercise.
3. Relax the muscles around those vertebrae (slump in the chair).

4. Lift and straighten your whole upper body by contracting the muscles around those vertebrae. Don't use any other muscles of your upper body. Allow the muscles of your lower vertebrae to do the movement, unaided by other parts of your back. If you have trouble isolating these specific muscles, keep moving your spine until you feel those muscles and vertebrae moving beneath your hand. Then try to move those muscles without moving any other part of your spine. Be patient; try this at different times on different days until you succeed in isolating the muscles of the lowest part of the back.

5. Continue to alternately relax and contract the muscles around these vertebrae so that you have a fluid, rocking motion in your lower back that alternately lifts and then releases your upper body.

6. Relax and feel what the movement has done.

Another way to describe this exercise:

1. Tuck your pelvis forward from your lower back. If you have done this correctly, your spine will be curved in the shape of a bow. This corresponds to the "slumping" position in step 3 above.

2. Move your pelvis backward, arching your back. This corresponds to step 4, in which you lift your upper body.

There is some difference in emphasis between the two instructions for the Pelvic Rock, but the motion of the pelvis forward and back is the same. Try doing this during long car trips and notice that it significantly eases lower back strain.

Leg Rotation in Different Directions

1. Sit comfortably in a chair, back far enough so that your feet don't quite reach the floor. This may be impossible for you if you have long legs. Perhaps you could put pillows on the

seat to raise yourself enough, but if not, try the exercise even if your feet reach the floor.

2. Knees together, rotate your lower legs around your knees so that your legs are moving together in the same direction, both of them making a circle to the right.
3. Change direction and rotate both legs together to the left.
4. Separate your knees a little and begin to rotate your lower legs in opposite directions so that each leg moves away from the other as it rotates.
5. Return to rotating your legs in the same direction, first to the right and then to the left, and then rotate your legs in the opposite direction from each other. Notice the differences in ease of movement from the first time you did this.
6. For a final challenge, rotate your ankles at the same time that you rotate your lower legs in the same and different directions.
7. Stop and feel what the movement has done.

Relational, or Self-Nurturing, Movements. These are movements in which you set up a relationship between one part of your body and another so that one part of the body can be felt as attending to or administering care to another part, which receives the support. As in the body awareness movements in the preceding subsection, the focus of your attention is your body sensations. When your attention wanders to other things, like a task you must finish or judgments about the movements you are doing, gently return your attention to the sensations of your body, including the feeling of your breath going in and out.

Massaging the Chest

1. Sit comfortably in a chair, with relaxed arms, legs, and spine. Breathe normally for several breaths, allowing your breath to deepen naturally as you relax.
2. Put one of your hands on your chest and one on your diaphragm and begin to gently explore your upper body as if you were completely unfamiliar with what it is. Move your fingertips over your skin or clothes and become aware of

what lies under each palm, each fingertip. Feel the dips and hills of your chest, the soft places, the hard places, the texture of the skin or clothing.

3. As you continue to move your hands over your chest and diaphragm, switch your focus so that you become your body being massaged by your hands. How do you feel about the touch of this person? Does this person care about you? Is this someone you would trust with your body? Feel the exploring, maybe even comforting, quality of your fingers on your upper body. Feel the physical touch of each of your fingers. Feel what each finger does, how it runs over your skin, plucks or circles your clothes, your bones.

4. Focus again on the fingers exploring the chest and diaphragm. Feel the dips and hills of your upper body, the texture of your clothes.

5. Focus again on your upper body, feeling the touch of your own fingers.

6. Stop and feel what you've done.

Knees from Side to Side

1. Sit comfortably on a chair with your feet on the floor, your knees together, and your arms comfortably in your lap. You may want to put a pillow behind you so that your feet can reach the floor when you are resting against the back of the chair.

2. With your knees together, move your bent legs from side to side, from right to left and back again. What is important in this exercise is that your *knees* lead the motion and that your hips follow rather than the other way around. Move your knees *before* you feel your hips move. That way, you can be sure your knees are leading and your hips are relaxing. If this is difficult for you, try moving just one leg at a time. Move one knee to the other side, then follow with the other knee. At first, you may move just a little bit from side to side. After you feel comfortable with the movement, you can allow your knees to stretch as far as they will go when

they move to each side. But don't push your knees or exert control of any kind; just move your knees from side to side, sensitive to the comfort level of your hips.

3. Stop and feel what the movement has done.

Passive Knee, Active Knee

1. Still sitting with your knees bent and feet apart, cross one knee over the other. Relax the upper leg completely. Move the lower leg from side to side, as you did during the last movement, so that the lower leg is giving the upper leg a ride. Let the upper leg relax and enjoy the support the lower leg is giving it as your legs move from side to side. Feel one leg work while the other leg relaxes and depends on the efforts of the first leg.

2. Now switch legs. The leg that worked before now relaxes over the knee of the other leg, and the leg that got a ride before now works. Is there any difference between the two legs in their willingness to work? To relax?

3. Now switch the legs again and notice any changes that occur in either leg's ability to work or relax.

4. Now switch again. After switching back and forth between each leg's being the worker and being the rider for five to ten minutes, stop and feel what the movement has done.

Head/Shoulder Dance

1. Sit in a comfortable chair with your feet on the floor (or rungs of a chair). Support your back against the back of the chair. Rest your hands on your thighs or in your lap. Take a few deep breaths and notice where your chest, shoulders, and neck feel tense or tight.

2. Rotate your left shoulder in small circles, changing to forward or backward motion from time to time. Your hands continue to rest on your knees or thighs. As you rotate, notice how your left shoulder comes up toward your ear and moves away from your ear.

3. After your shoulder rotation is well established, slowly

move your head from side to side at the same time that you rotate your left shoulder, leading the motion with your chin so that your neck muscles are making very little effort to turn your head. Move the focus of your attention from chest to shoulder to neck and back again. Notice any sense of loosening that results from these distinctions you are increasingly aware of between your upper body parts. Feel these as separate parts. After a few minutes, stop the movements and feel what you've done. Notice the difference between the two sides of your upper body.

4. Rotate your right shoulder in small circles, changing to forward or backward motion from time to time. Your hands continue to rest on your knees or thighs. As you rotate, notice how your right shoulder comes up toward your ear and moves away from your ear. After a few minutes, stop your shoulder rotations and feel what you've done.

5. After your shoulder rotation is well established, slowly move your head from side to side at the same time that you rotate your right shoulder, leading the motion with your chin so that your neck muscles are making very little effort to turn your head. Move the focus of your attention from chest to shoulder to neck and back again. Notice any sense of loosening that results from these distinctions you are increasingly aware of between your upper body parts. Feel these as separate parts. After a few minutes, stop the movements and feel what you've done.

The movements suggested in this subsection have been adapted specifically for sitting in a chair or half-sitting on a couch so that you can do them while reading this book. If you find these sitting movements soothing, it may be that you would find it even more relaxing to do similar movements while lying down on a comfortable mat and following the directions on an audiocassette. For ordering instructions, see the form in the back of the book.

Using Everyday Movements to Feel Your Body

Over the long run, the most effective exercises you will do are the ordinary movements you perform in your everyday life. Why not work on healing your body twenty-four hours a day instead of during just one hour of a formal exercise session? After all, you have to move around anyway; you might as well move in a way that enhances rather than compromises your well-being. In order to begin moving in a way that promotes your ease and/or healing, you need to start feeling how your everyday movements affect your body.

After having arthritis for several years, I spent a summer on the staff of a resort in Big Sur. Since I was in meetings most of the day, I wanted to make certain I had a period of vigorous exercise in the mornings. I therefore requested the job of cabin cleaning, a daily three-hour stint of preparing cabins for new guests. Usually only teenagers were assigned to cabin cleaning because of the prevailing belief that the job required youth and stamina. The duties were clear-cut: replace the sheets, blankets, and bedspreads on every bed; sweep the floors; scour the sinks and toilets; empty the trash; and wash the windows and mirrors. The tasks were performed at high speed because anywhere from fifteen to twenty-five cabins needed to be done by lunchtime.

Because this job required no conceptual thinking, I spent the entire work period every day as an exercise session, interweaving my movements and the contact I had with inanimate objects. It required particular intimacy between my body and my task. I bent and stretched my back while changing the bed linens; I twisted my body rhythmically to sweep the floors; I hung sequentially from each vertebra to scour the toilets; I squeezed the Windex bottle with all five fingers, alternating my hands, to wash the windows. I breathed fully and deeply to set a rhythm for my body movements.

After a few weeks of this activity, I was exhilarated and bursting with energy. My posture had improved dramatically from changing twenty to forty beds each morning. In contrast, by lunchtime every day, almost all of my coworkers (none over twenty-five and most in their teens) would be complaining about their backaches from making so many beds and scouring all those sinks. I still marvel at the efficacy of my exercises—not only the physicality of them but the difference it made in my sense of well-being and my stamina to be so intimately connected with my activity.

One morning as I was washing windows, the group leader came by. She was a good friend and knew that I was likely to be doing my work from my body's point of view. As she watched me squeezing my Windex bottle, she started laughing and said, "I know you're doing hand exercises, Darlene, but couldn't you wash the windows a little, too?" I suddenly realized that squeezing a nearly empty Windex bottle almost a hundred times before I got any Windex on the window was an unacceptable speed at which to get any window washing done. I was so focused on my exercises that I had lost sight of my work! I don't advocate concentrating on your body's movements to the detriment of your work, but I do want to suggest that you can become very good at doing both.

You can practice living from the point of view of your body every day in your workaday life. You can choose to take the body's point of view for a few hours a day, a few days a week, a few months at a time, a year, or as a more or less permanent point of view for the rest of your life. I encourage you to try it as an experiment. At the very least, you will increase your mental agility by shifting back and forth from goal-directed thinking and decision making to registering feelings and sensations from different parts of your body. You may find that cerebral functions such as thinking and decision making become clearer and easier once you pay attention to your body. That is because you will have a stable viewpoint from which to judge your possibilities.

When we feel settled in our bodies, we frequently experience a clarity and certainty that are very helpful in arranging the priorities of our ordinary lives. When we become proficient at taking our bodies' point of view as we move through our daily lives, we will have honed a powerful tool for being intimately connected to The One Who Is Not Busy.

STRATEGIES FOR MANAGING PHYSICAL PAIN

There are some actual physical movements that are helpful in relieving certain kinds of pain. The following have been published before in my book *Arthritis: Stop Suffering, Start Moving/ Everyday Exercises for Body and Mind*. I recommend that book as a manual for living with chronic pain and using the movements you do to accomplish your daily chores in such a way as to ease that pain.

You can use various strategies to lessen or eliminate pain during movement. When you feel pain while exercising or while moving around doing your everyday tasks, you have the opportunity to use your pain as a guide to deeper penetration of your muscles and nerves, to moving or relaxing in such a way that the pain is affected directly by what you do. Never ignore pain. The presence of pain is an opportunity to learn conscious living so thoroughly that it informs your whole life and your outlook, beyond your physical movements. If you feel discomfort or pain while exercising or doing some physical task, like vacuuming or cooking, immediately experiment with variations in your movements to see what does what to the pain. Try the following strategies:

1. *Do less of the movement that is hurting you.* If you are mixing ingredients in a large bowl, making large circles with your arm to blend the mixture with a spoon, make your arm circles smaller. Or perform only a portion of the circle, gently folding small amounts of the mixture over itself, so that your arm moves back and forth a small distance along the path of your large motion. If you are walking, take smaller steps for a few minutes, then return to your usual stride to see whether that made any difference. If you are lifting dishes to the cupboard, lighten your load. Lift a dish or two at a time. This emphasizes the motions rather than the load, which should be helpful to your muscles and joints. You may find that doing a much smaller movement for a little while will enable you to resume the larger movement.

If the pain persists after you return to the larger movement, move your arm on the "frontier" of your pain, the area where movement just begins to be painful but is not quite painful yet. If you move into this area—but stop short of causing real pain—you may expand the area of comfort to include much more of the originally painful movement. In other words, you reduce the amount of territory occupied by pain.

Expanding your area of comfort in one situation (your exercise session, for instance) often means you will have expanded it generally, in other situations as well. It's as if your brain discovers that there is actually more space in your body to do that movement than it originally thought—because you slowed down enough to demonstrate that very thoroughly to your brain.

2. *Do a different movement than the one that is hurting you.* Moving in a different direction or dimension is often effective in stretching the joint or releasing the muscle just enough to get the little bit of space in the joint or muscle that was needed to eliminate discomfort. If it hurts to move your arm up and down to reach for something on the shelf, try moving it gently across your body a few times, or letting your hand rotate your arm in your shoulder socket as it hangs at your side. Rotation is especially good because it moves the painful area in all directions. Then you can return to the original motion—that is, reaching the shelf—and see whether you have reduced or eliminated the pain.

3. *Massage the painful area.* If you have been walking for a while in the park and your ankles start to ache, sit down on a bench, lift each ankle to your knee, and gently massage the painful and/ or swollen areas. If you can succeed in reducing the swelling by gently pinching and rubbing the swollen areas, when you get back onto your feet, you will feel much, much better. If you have been sitting for a while at your desk and your hip "catches" when you suddenly rise, causing you to gasp with pain, you can beat on your hip area gently with your fists and loosen it enough to take steps without discomfort. What is required to minister to yourself in this way is some sense that whatever discomfort you feel, you can take care of it yourself.

4. *Passively move the painful area with a part more distal to it.* Even if your joints are usually very painful with movement, they can often be moved painlessly if someone else does the moving. Passive movement is an enormously effective technique for relaxing muscles and increasing mobility in the joints. This makes it ideal for pain relief.

Any body part that is close to the torso can be moved by another part that is farther from the torso. For instance, if your hips hurt, your bent knees moving gently together from side to side can relax and soothe your hips. If your shoulder hurts, your hand moving your straight arm around your shoulder can ease the shoulder gently into a more comfortable position. If your neck hurts, moving the very top of your head in a small circular motion will relax your neck muscles.

In order to become skilled at relieving one part of your body by moving another, more distal, part, you need to learn how to move different parts of your body independently from each other. If you want to relieve a sore hip by moving your leg, you need to feel your hip muscles relaxing and gently being moved by the active movement of your leg. Developing this skill takes practice as well as concentration on what body parts you are attempting to isolate with your movement. If you have difficulty at first determining what part of you is actively moving and what part is being passively moved, ask someone to help you. Your friend can move your leg for you while you concentrate on relaxing your hip; this will let you know what it feels like for your hip to be passively moved. Then you can move your leg so as to duplicate the feeling you had in your hip when your friend was moving your leg. In this way, you can learn how to ease your own pain by moving different parts of your body in relation to each other.

5. *With your breath, create an inner landscape so wide that your path of movement always bypasses pain.* This is a sophisticated strategy, learned and perfected over a long period of time. This state of mind is what might develop from employing the preceding four strategies whenever you have pain. From how you move and breathe, your body/brain somehow learns what is required to

live a relatively pain-free existence. Your body/brain puts together all the information you have been gathering during your
exercise periods and your daily life movements and comes up
with solutions you could not have managed consciously. This is
the potential of the storehouse of information you have gathered
by attending to the sensations of your body—those of discomfort,
pleasure, and ease. When you can return to this state of mind
every day, or even a few times a week, the activities you wish to
do will be much less limited by chronic pain.

You must be consistent about employing these techniques and
remind yourself of what is important in any particular situation:
is it more important to get dinner on the stove right this minute
or to reduce your pain level now? You know that in all cases,
your health and comfort are more important. Stop and do a few
loosening movements and get dinner on the stove three or four
minutes later. When you stop working and address your pain
right when it's happening, not only do you ease it then, but you
are breaking the habit of pain itself. You are interrupting your
usual mind-set of assuming that getting dinner ready will be accompanied by pain. Stop putting up with pain! Start demanding
of yourself that you put your own comfort level and healing potential ahead of the efficient completion of mundane tasks.
Whenever it hurts, stop and take the opportunity to teach yourself how to move without hurting. You are investing in a pain-free
future.

9

CONNECTION

Turning Suffering Inside Out

❧ ❧

LIBERATION from the painful, unsatisfying habits of aversion and clinging lies in developing the intimate connections that sustain our human life.

CONNECTION AND ALIENATION

I've come to think that alienation, lack of connection, is our greatest suffering: our separation from each other, from the earth, from our own bodies, from our feelings and emotions, from our creativity, and from our activity itself. This alienation is very pervasive right now in our culture. We all feel this estrangement, reflected in the unraveling of the fabric of our society, in which very few individuals feel any responsibility for our collective well-being. It isn't only minority groups who must struggle for full acceptance politically and economically and who feel ill-treated and left out of the so-called mainstream; almost everybody, regardless of privilege or opportunity, feels dismissed, unheeded, unlistened to. People don't talk to each other; they call their lawyers.

In many ways, how we live our lives today weakens or threatens the fundamental connections that we as human beings have enjoyed since ancient times. Despite what generations of our ancestors knew, we need a clock to tell what time it is, a therapist to help us discover our feelings, machines to exercise our bodies, money to buy food, and science to explain processes that we probably once understood as intimately as our own breath.

We may be able to function adequately under these conditions day to day, but when we fall into dire situations, we are overwhelmed by our misery because we have lost the connections that contribute to our well-being as humans—the primal, healing connections to:

- *Our bodies and their sensations:* This includes the rhythm of our breathing.
- *Our sensory reality, the constant stream of sensory input:* This includes what we see as we look around a room, the sounds that constitute the comforting, contextual background noise of our lives to which we usually pay no conscious attention.
- *Our yearnings and needs:* Because emotional needs—such as the need to grieve a great loss for as long as a year or to perform some ceremony or ritual that satisfies deep, inchoate feelings that don't make sense—often seem irrational, our linear, material culture simply overlooks them as nonexistent or discounts them as silly, even indulgent.
- *Our feelings and emotions:* We learn early that all but the mildest feelings are considered socially inappropriate, and our real feelings may be painfully sad or dangerously angry.
- *Our creativity:* As we grow up and make a great effort to do what we think we should do and get everything done on time, we may gradually lose touch with our creative energies, the ability to think in an original way. Such regimentation may even affect our sexuality, an extension of our creative life.
- *Our fellow beings:* If we devote most of our waking time to work and the maintenance of our "lifestyle" instead of spending some unstructured time with friends and family members, our connections to our fellow beings degenerate into superficial associations rather than intimate, affectionate relationships that offer real support in times of need.
- *Our activity itself:* Most profoundly tragic, we have lost our

connection to the movements that we make every moment in the course of a day. After a day of work, we arrive home exhausted, needing refreshment, whereas a true involvement in our activity could have energized and challenged us.

When we lose these all-important primal connections, or never really establish them in the first place, then we have no safety net to catch us when we get knocked off balance by stress or catastrophe. We're not anchored by any rich net of affiliations to start with, so when everything comes apart, we get confused about our priorities, our values, what is really most important to us. We start running to the doctor, listening to the TV talk show, writing the advice columnist, frantically consulting supposed experts, instead of turning to the only real source of personal wisdom—our own hearts—because we can't find our hearts.

Denial and Resignation

Next to our various addictions, our society's favorite coping mechanism is denial: insulation from body, pain, the natural world, old age, death, feeling, and emotion. We are so deluged with information about the suffering of people all over the world that many of us recoil from suffering of any kind. Some of us avoid the news and the sights of the street, habitually turning away from homeless people, not out of meanness but as self-protection. We don't want to deal with incidental suffering, the suffering that is simply part of going about our business. We become insular, narrowing our world and concerns to just our lives, our loved ones, our personal pursuits. People who have the necessary financial resources sometimes become quite successful at avoiding really gross forms of suffering. I don't blame people for keeping suffering at bay if they can; it's such a reflexive thing to do. But I think there's a price to be paid for such insulation.

Since feelings, pain, and fear of death arise in the body, denying them allows us to lead our lives from our heads. Many of us use our bodies just to get our brains from place to place. Some of us spend a lot of time buffing up, shaping our bodies in the gym, and increasing our heart rate. Our culture turns out gorgeous old people who run marathons, but this still is not necessarily inhabiting the body. It's more like viewing the body as an art form, sculpting it to fit our mental ideals. Our bodies, with their desires and emotions, can be scary to actually inhabit. Living from the point of view of our bodies, accepting their fate as our fate, aware of ourselves as muscle and bone and nerve cell, we are eerily aware of our mortality.

In the short term, denial can be very useful. It can get us through deadlines and important milestones that getting in touch with our feelings of resistance and pain might hinder, just as an athlete finishes a marathon regardless of her pain. When people told me I couldn't go white-water rafting because of my arthritis, I denied my disability. Why couldn't I do what any able-bodied person could? If I had "accepted" my restrictions, I wouldn't have had so much fun. So denial can be handy in the short term.

But if denial is used habitually as a long-term strategy to deal with adversity, eventually it robs our lives of their interest and vitality. To stay in denial, we must cut off all feeling and sensation arising from our bodies and our emotions. Information about the direness of our situation is exactly what we are trying to avoid. So we can't allow any feeling to come up from our gut. Nor can we allow any information to enter from the outside, like a friend seeing us and saying, "Oh, you look so tired today! Can I help you with something?" We say, "No, no," annoyed rather than comforted by our friend's concern. We cut off our bodily feelings; we dismiss our friend.

To remain in denial, we must cut off more and more external feedback until our world is extremely narrow and bleak. We come to live in some tiny strip of consciousness, maybe just what is needed to get up, go to work, come home, park ourselves in front of the TV, go to bed. We can't have any intimate interactions because we can't afford experiences that would cause feeling to break through our denial, like relaxing, playing, sinking into our bodies, exciting our feelings. If we persist in shutting out any evidence of our pain or fear, we eventually come to exist on narrow, bleak little tundras of our own creation. Is this a life worth living?

The opposite extreme is resignation or victimhood. When faced with a catastrophic situation, we cry out, "Why me?" and go to bed and pull the covers over our heads. We refuse to entertain any solution to our suffering. We get caught up in being a victim, afraid to risk any engagement with our situation. Indeed, there's not enough energy in this strategy to consider any possibility of change. We become totally passive, resigned. Nothing a friend or doctor suggests can possibly help. We give up our lives to loss.

Like denial, resignation is great in the short term. We all occasionally need what the corporate world calls a "mental health day." We call in sick to work, curl up in bed with potato chips and cookies, and watch daytime TV. A day of this kind of comforting distraction is usually enough to refresh and rejuvenate most of us. The next day, we go back to work, prepared to reengage. It is a wise and productive worker who occasionally treats herself to this needed break in routine. But long-term, such passivity becomes draining rather than refreshing. We lose more and more energy and self-determination until we are unable to summon the will and courage to engage effectively with the sources of our suffering.

Sometimes after a lecture in which I have told the story of my efforts to deal with rheumatoid arthritis, someone will come up and tell me that he or she has a friend or relative in a similar situation—exhausted by pain or experiencing paralysis or loss of mobility from a disease or an injury. The concerned friend implores me to see the person, emphasizing his or her desperate condition. I always agree. For me, people in this kind of dire circumstance are my peers, my compadres. It is not unusual, however, for a month or two to pass and the desperate person never appears. The friend calls me, puzzled and sad, explaining that even though he or she impressed upon the loved one the accessibility of my approach, the person remains bedridden or resigned to suffering: "Maybe it could help her, but not me."

Although the concerned friend is usually bewildered, I actually understand. If you are in great pain, barely functioning, miserable, and hopeless, and someone tells you there is a possibility of relief if you will only make the effort, you are not necessarily relieved to hear this. Instead, you may be very conflicted. Committing yourself to a potential solution involves coming into feeling: feeling how much pain you are actually in (rather than minimizing it to yourself, which has become your habit); feeling how desperate you really are (If this goes on too much longer, I will want to die); and potentially most devastating, risking that the effort you make will result in improvement, that it will actually be your solution, your cure, rather than just raising your hopes only to reconfirm your hopeless position later. That is the most dangerous thought of all, making that investment. If you are resigned to the inevitability of your misery, coming into your feelings about it is perilous indeed.

The trouble with both denial and resignation is that there's not enough energy in either one of them to make them effective long-term strategies for coping with pain and stress. To make decisions that reflect our values and the direction in which we must go to solve our problems, we need every piece of information that denial deprives us of. To craft a strategy to meet the demands of tremendous pressure at work or a sudden catastrophe at home, we need access to all our ingenuity, creativity, and wisdom, which is exactly what becoming a victim robs us of.

So if neither denial nor resignation works as a strategy for dealing with stress and pain, what *is* effective?

REESTABLISHING THE PRIMAL CONNECTIONS

Whereas the feeling of alienation may be our greatest suffering, its opposite—connection, a sense of union or intimacy—may be our greatest comfort and joy. All the gifts of healing I learned from my pain have to do with reestablishing these primal, healing connections.

To Our Body and Breath

Before I was stricken with my disease, I only knew my body from the outside, how it looked in a mirror. Despite its being strong and young and dependable, I was very critical of it. Too much fat over here, legs too short for my long torso, shoulders too broad for my small frame. I would never appear in short shorts because the shape of my knees fell well below beauty queen standards, and I didn't wish to impose my physical flaws on others. (Mostly, I didn't want to be judged for them!) The idea that I might ever cavort about in short shorts because it's hot out and be unconcerned with how people might judge my artificially round, arthritic knees, scarred from replacement surgery, was unthinkable. What changed is that I'm no longer just an observer. Now I can't tell exactly where my body ends and what I mysteriously refer to as "I" begins. My body and its sensations are how I experience my reality. My breath sets a rhythm for my activity. I breathe in the world, then I breathe it out. I feel my body's yearnings as the wellspring of my own desire. Grounded in my body, I am able to distinguish between generosity and obligation, need and avarice, appetite and obsession.

I also have learned to love to move, both minutely and vigorously. I have come to understand that movement is one of my body's yearnings. Movement is what bodies, composed of muscle and nerve fiber, yearn to do. I no longer take movement for granted; I slide into it, luxuriate in it, experience it as a tremendous enrichment of my life, through my body, expanding my horizons with my breath.

To Our Deep Yearnings and Needs

More subtle than bodily cravings, the need for creativity and self-expression must have some sort of spacious playing field to be felt and cultivated. Although we all yearn to play and create, most of us don't take those impulses seriously and regard their satisfaction as important for our health and balance. I have come to recognize that expressing my urge to create—whether producing some material product, having sex, solving a problem, devising, inventing, or playing—makes a tremendous contribution to my health. Thus, I have set up a work pattern that encourages the flow of my own particular stream of original thought: relaxation; intense, short work periods without distraction; frequent breaks—all of which encourage me to cultivate the practice of playing with thoughts and feelings and the obstacles that block my path.

While I have been writing this book, my rheumatoid arthritis has virtually gone into remission, a reminder to me of how important it is to my well-being to set aside time in my day to express some sort of creative impulse. I have had clients who came to me with chronic physical problems that I felt intuitively were related to their inability for whatever reason to find some creative outlet for their energies. It felt to me as if their organic vitality were somehow working against the tissue in their bodies, as an autoimmune disease does, rather than flowing out into the world through their hands and minds. Jesus reputedly said that if you don't express what is in you, what is in you will destroy you. I don't think most of us take our yearnings for self-expression seriously enough to include that need in our day-to-day lives.

Admittedly, it might be very hard to turn a job at Burger King into some sort of ultimate self-fulfillment, but the wish to do so is very close to the yearning to live wholeheartedly, with our full being, which can be indulged anywhere. When I was an office temp, I used to amuse myself by creating elegant letters with aesthetically pleasing proportions and borders from the dictation I took. A few of my various bosses told me it actually gave them pleasure to sign such a distinctive page. It saved me from stupefaction.

To Our Feelings

From my study of Zen meditation, I have learned to practice respect for all my feelings: anxiety, pain, hatred, pettiness, sympathy, resistance, joy. Every one is sacred; none is inherently less real than another. By myself and with friends, I have developed rituals that allow safe connection with feelings of despair, bitterness, grief. We've acknowledged the end of menses, the loss of a beloved brother, and the finding of a birth mother this way. When we practice these rituals together, expressing intense feelings through motions that employ objects used for such purpose since the beginning of time—candles, plants, incense, stones, drums—the shared activity is imbued with a gravity and release that can't be accounted for by the simplicity of the objects and motions involved. I think the powerful healing effect of these simple observances is often due merely to the fact that we've taken our feelings seriously enough to create a little ceremony to express them.

A client of mine became very annoyed and scolded her husband for coming in and telling me a joke while I was massaging her at her house. When I asked why she minded so much, she said, "He was using up my time with you." She was not in a state of mind that could be satisfied by simply listening to the sound of her husband's voice as he told a joke, feeling my fingers on her body, and sensing the animal presence of the three of us sharing the room. She didn't even examine the starved, jealous mind that resented his brief interruption.

Paradoxically, noticing this kind of small-mindedness can actually add rich texture to the weave of your life. When you include the shadow in your perceptions, your conscious life begins to be shaded and textured by your anguish and petty snits. Sanitizing your thoughts and preoccupations not only squanders vital energy that would be better spent in your creative endeavors, but your not-so-presentable life can be enormously enriching and provide the compost for the development of compassion. If you have never given in to temptation of any kind, how can you ever understand—or embrace—the sinner? I pointed out some of these things to my client. The next time I saw her, she told me that after our session, she had begun to be flooded with perceptions. She had noticed how much pain her tense relationship with her teenage son was causing her. Being numb had enabled her to tolerate their friction, but now it was clear to her that she could no longer live with those hard feelings. She had to engage him and discuss their problems.

People sometimes ask me where my own healing energy comes from. How, in the midst of this pain, this implacable slow crippling, can I encourage myself and other people? My answer is that my healing comes from my bitterness itself, my despair, my terror. It comes from the shadow. I dip down into that muck again and again and then am flooded with its healing energy. Despite the renewal and vitality I get from facing my deepest fears, I don't go willingly when they call. I've been around that wheel a million times: first, I feel the despair, but I deny it for a few days; then, its tugs become more insistent in proportion to my resistance; finally, it overwhelms me and pulls me down, kicking and screaming all the way. It's clear I am caught, so at last I give up to this reunion with the dark aspect of my adjustment to pain and loss. Immediately, the release begins: first peace, then the flood of vitality and healing energy.

I can never simply give up to my despair when I first feel it stir. You'd think after a million times with a happy ending, I could give up right away and just say, "Take me, I'm yours," but I never can. I always resist. I guess that's why it's called despair. If you went willingly, it would be called something hopeful, like purification or renewal. It's staring defeat and annihilation in the face that's so terrifying; I must resist until it overwhelms me. But I've come to trust it deeply. It's enriched my life, informed my work, and taught me not to fear the dark.

To Other People

One aspect of intimacy that particularly interests me is relationship with other people, specifically the kind of relationship that promotes healing and nurtures your ability to see things as they are. I advocate consciously developing nurturing relationships: making the kind of intimate connection with others in which "I" and "thou," "otherness," disappears, or enough of the "otherness" disappears that what you feel is the connection, not the otherness. Although these relationships are not only with people, the ones with people are certainly the most problematic and revealing. Other people help you to see the conflict between what you want and the way life really is. In that gap, your life becomes alive and compelling. When I became ill, I gave up self-sufficiency, my illusion of myself as an independent, self-reliant, strong woman. I didn't expect it, but I got something in exchange: relationship. All the difficulties you have with other people give you a tremendous opportunity for intimacy if you and they are willing to process difficult feelings.

As Joko Beck points out in *Everyday Zen:*

> Relationships with people, especially close and trusting ones, are our best way to grow. In them we can see what our mind, our body, our senses, and our thoughts really are. There is no way that is superior to relationships in helping us see where we're stuck and what we're holding onto. As long as our buttons are pushed, we have a great chance to learn and grow. So a relationship is a great gift not because it makes us happy—it often doesn't—but because any intimate relationship, if we view it as practice, is the clearest mirror we can find. If we understand zazen and our practice, we can begin to get acquainted with ourselves and how our troublesome emotions wreak havoc with our lives. Observing our relationships illuminates our activity: puts a searchlight on our unkind thoughts about people and situations. We must make conscious how terrible we think someone is or how terrible we are, what we want, what we expect, the cloud over everything.

If you are sick or under a lot of stress, your family and friends might unintentionally isolate you, thinking they are protecting you from additional stress, when actually they are cutting you off from their lives. If you're sick, your daughter may not share with you her fear of being ostracized if she refuses to take drugs with schoolmates; your friends may not tell you about their concerns anymore, thinking they are trivial compared to your problems; your husband may not "bother" you with his financial worries.

However, when you feel so isolated by your pain or stress, what you yearn for is to be included, reassured that you are still connected with people. Because those around you feel so helpless in the face of your ordeal, it is usually up to you to make the first move, to proclaim your need to be included, not protected, if that's how you feel.

Research tells us that tending to others and sharing their suffering may have an ameliorating effect on our own. I have a friend who was terribly abused as a child and has suffered a great deal in her life. She studied to become an acupuncturist and has been working with patients in San Francisco. Even though she has been virtually penniless at times and has no economic security of her own, she volunteered recently to go to Mexico and work in a clinic there, just for room and board. When I commented on how altruistic this seemed, she said candidly, "The only way I ever found to deal with my own suffering is to attend to the suffering of other people."

To the Activity of Our Daily Lives

I consider it the greatest tragedy of our modern life that we spend all day doing a job but are so disconnected from our activity itself that we do not even notice what we're doing. Since we often find our jobs deadening and exhausting, we come home and need the evenings, and then the weekends, to recover from the way we spend our days. Spending most of our lives this way is sad, indeed. We think the only way we can get through our work-week is to numb ourselves, but actually the opposite is true. We need to wake up, to be alive and involved in our activity, to live all our moments, to do each thing for the sake of doing it. I know many people who believe the solution to work as boredom is to get a "meaningful" job, one that holds inherent interest, so that they are either fulfilling themselves through it or doing good for others. I don't think this is necessary, however. We need not replace what we do for a living with a "meaningful" job (thank God); we only need to connect with our activity, to notice it, to stop dismissing it as mundane and then going numb.

I had a favorite client, Julia, who came to me once a week for years for treatment for her rheumatoid arthritis. Due to the massage and movement sessions with me and her own exercises between treatments, Julia was very high-functioning. She had a full-time job and a family. She was capable of relaxing—she became a noodle on the massage table—but the minute her session was over, she would jump up and start putting on her clothes so frantically, she would undo everything she had just done in the realm of stretching her joints. I could never successfully communicate to her this idea of using her daily life as one long exercise in healing. And it became apparent over the months that that was the only thing that would really make a difference in her level of health. Then one night she said to me as she was rushing out the door after her session, "I hate when you give me new exercises." I was quite surprised. "You do?" I said.

"I get up in the morning, go to work, work all day, come home, fix dinner, eat dinner, clean up dinner, and by then it's eight o'clock," she explained. "I have maybe two hours, tops, to live my own life, to really be alive. Whenever you give me new relaxation exercises, I have to do my work twice as fast and do my exercises as fast as I can so that I can have some time for myself."

So I said, "Julia, weren't you alive when you went to work? When you came home and fixed dinner, ate dinner, and so on? And weren't you alive especially when you did those relaxation self-awareness exercises I gave you for your pain?" "Oh, yeah," she replied sheepishly. And of course, we both realized what the problem was: she divided up her life into tasks she had to do and actual *living*, and she madly rushed through the mandatory tasks so that she could begin to live. She defined being alive as having unstructured time, time that belonged only to her, when she was free of obligation. Unfortunately for her—and for most of us— that kind of free time is quite rare. If we define really being alive that way, we are going to be numb most of the time and thereby squander the vast majority of the precious time that we have to live. No wonder Julia felt, despite a supportive, loving family and three homes in different beautiful places in California, that she was a deprived person. No wonder she spent so much of her time contracting her muscles and compressing her joints.

Living is about active participation and total involvement in our everyday activity. Hanging out with the laundry, the dishes; fingering the uneven surface of a rock; feeling the evaporation of sweat on the back of our necks on a sultry summer afternoon, the comforting warmth of a cup of coffee or tea on a rainy evening, even the flash of irritation when someone cuts us off on the freeway. Our hearts start beating faster, our jaws clench in rage, we might say or think something dramatic. That may be the most alive we feel all day! We usually dismiss such events as mundane, but they are actually the stuff of our lives, and therefore our healing.

Healing for me is connection to my activity itself, the practice of doing each thing for its own sake, and of course, intimacy with other people, plants, the earth and sky, the laundry, the traffic, the commercials, the mundane anguish of daily existence. There's nothing special or tragic about it; it's just my life, day in and day out. Even though our lives are nothing special, it's not easy to penetrate our numbness and become willing to open ourselves up to all the details of our daily lives, including the stress and pain. Because of our conditioning to avoid unpleasantness, the hardest thing may not be bearing the unpleasant experiences we have so much as learning how to experience the details of our suffering so thoroughly that "suffering," "stress," and "pain" lose their distinctive character and just become our lives, and rich lives at that. We're usually so caught up in our opinions that we can't experience things as they are. We'd rather think about how "unfair" something is, or how morally superior we ourselves are, than experience the actual feelings involved in a disappointment at work. But how we open ourselves to feeling, how we embrace all the experiences life has to offer, has a great deal to do with how connected we feel.

To Our Suffering

I think our connections to people and things are shaped by our relationship to our suffering. I actually know of no better way to deal with pain and suffering than intimacy with it. By intimacy, I mean allowing ourselves to feel the actual experience of suffering, discomfort, anguish, distress, despair. Absorbing and being the suffering. And if we cannot absorb and be it, then settling into the painful isolation of not absorbing and not being it. This, too, is the intimacy of suffering. This is not passivity or nonaction; instead, it is action from a state of complete acceptance. Simply being the suffering. Complete openness, complete vulnerability to life. This might go on at the same time as we are railing against our pain and searching for ways to stop it. Completely accepting our suffering and looking for ways to end it don't hinder each other. They are both active encounters with our lives.

We must begin by cultivating the ability to acknowledge our own suffering and that of others. To quote from a lecture given by Norman Fischer, abbot of the San Francisco Zen Center:

> We are human beings, and we must feel love and hate, elation and terrible grief. But underneath these things, we come to see, through our practice, there is a wider world beyond our concerns—a wild, radically sane world, in which we can accept what occurs, aware of our feelings of grief or happiness, but not pushed around by them. This kind of acceptance does not mean not caring. In fact with this real total acceptance comes a transformation in our ability to care—we care for everything very deeply. Not just victims, not just suffering people, but all people and not just all people, but also animals and plants and also for ourselves.

The world that opened to me through engaging the physical suffering and mental anguish caused by my disease has turned out to be inexpressibly rich. Because if we can engage with our suffering—connect with it, dance with it, tease it, coax it, curse it, as well as trying to change it, just consider it our lives, experience it as our lives, the only lives we have—it changes the quality of that suffering. It's not just our suffering; it's everything. When we look at it that way, we can't make the usual divisions. We feel connected with everything. It's strangely comforting—paradoxically comforting. In the moment that we can embrace our own suffering, the barrier between ourselves and others is gone.

I started observing the healing effect that connection had on me for the first time when I was very ill. I felt an intimacy I had never before noticed with my body and breath and their movements and fluctuations, their yearnings; I felt deeply aware of my needs, how each need demands its own gratification and specifically what the cost of ignoring each need is. Experiencing the connection to my feelings, the sacredness of each one, I came to understand that all feelings—petty feelings, keeping track of who last did the dishes; and generous feelings, offering help with no thought of holding back—have equal value from the point of view of living life thoroughly. Respect for all these feelings allows me to be connected with my suffering, to acknowledge it, to engage with it as a wellspring of vitality. And in fact, when I experience my pain that way—as one of the myriad feelings that come and go—I often fail to name it as suffering in particular; it's just my experience.

PART FOUR

RETURNING TO THE PRESENT MOMENT

10

PAYING ATTENTION

❦ ❧

THE technique that many of us use to become more conscious of the fundamental elements of our lives is meditation, which can be defined simply as awareness. There is an infinite variety of things to be aware of: our breath, body sensations, thoughts, moods, physical movements; the animal presence of other people in the room; the sounds we hear—to name a few. Or we might step back and look at the recurring patterns of any of these things, observing, for example, the way our minds organize incoming sense data, whether our body sensations are pleasant or unpleasant, whether our thoughts are random or repetitious. Or we might choose to be aware of all of these things at once, noticing whether our breathing is fast or slow, where our body is tense; observing how our attention is drawn to sounds that arise and then disappear; being aware of how sleepy we feel; remembering an argument we had earlier in the day.

Learning how to pay this kind of attention can radically change the quality of pain or stress because the kind of mind it produces is clear and focused compared to our usual churning, busy, jumbled mind. This lucid mind gives us a perspective from which we can set priorities in our lives based on our real values rather than mere habit. A great deal of our daily stress stems from confusion over what is really important to us. Do we actually need to get dinner on the table as fast as possible, or is that just a habit we could reevaluate? Could we take our time and make the dinner prep a creative and enjoyable experience? One in which we're also aware of our breath, our body's movements? Or our current feelings for the person who is helping us with the prep or perhaps instead watching TV in the next room? If hunger is really the motivation for rushing through dinner prep oblivious to our experience, could we munch carrots as we go? Do we really have to clean our whole house every Saturday, or could that be a totally free and unstructured day after 12:00 noon? It is good to become conscious of our actual values. We might really believe that our well-being is more important than living efficiently, but we might have forgotten our beliefs in the crush of daily demands.

So how do you begin to develop this ability to pay attention and use it to cultivate your healing, your sense of ease, your capacity to discover the happiness that is already there? You can start by tuning in to your five senses, your posture, and your breathing anytime. Now, for instance, notice how your body feels in your chair. Where are your feet placed? Your bottom? Your hands? Feel the muscles in your back: first the section of your spine above your sitting muscles, then the muscles nearer your waist, and finally the muscles of your upper back around your shoulderblades. Does one of these areas carry more tension than another? Does your chair support your upper body well, or do you feel the discomfort of tension along your neck and shoulders? Can you shift to relieve some of that tension? Notice whether moving your shoulders or turning your head to change the position of your neck while you read makes you feel more at ease.

Feel your breath expand and contract your diaphragm area. Can you just notice your breath without affecting its rhythm? How far into your body does the movement from the expansion and contraction of your diaphragm go? Are your shoulders moved by your breath? Is your chest moved by your breath? Or is movement pretty much confined to your diaphragm?

What can you see besides this page? Can you see parts of the room around the edges of the book? Is there a scent in the room that you may not have consciously noticed before? Someone's perfume? An animal? Wood smoke from a fire? Your own hair or clothes? Can you taste anything? Does some flavor linger from your last meal? What can you feel on the surface of your skin? The temperature of the air? Your clothes? Your jewelry? Your hair? Your eyeglasses? What is it you hear right now? A ventilation system? Music? Your neighbor's movements above you or next door? Passing cars? An airplane? Your refrigerator running? Close your eyes and notice all the sounds around you. This is your world, your sensory life right now. Including the sensations of the body and its various sense impressions adds rich texture to all the moments of your life.

It's easy to do this tuning-in exercise, this awareness meditation, while you're following my instruction in this book. But when you're on your feet, involved in getting something done, it's harder. You have to actually cultivate the skill to notice the world of breath and body in order to be able to go to it at will. Then you can use that awareness to penetrate the state of mind that gets wound up with the stress of a deadline or the despair you feel about your physical pain or disability. On the ordinary level of consciousness where you usually live, you have demands and expectations and no time. In the world of sensation that you've just visited, there is no time limit. It's boundless. That why there is no stress there. There may be different kinds of feelings, like peace or agitation, sadness or anger, but there's no pressure to be anything other than what you are.

Every day you can practice paying attention to the world in which you live this very moment. Sit still for twenty to thirty minutes and just notice your sensations, thoughts, and sense impressions. Practice noticing them without worrying about what they are. After some weeks of this sort of practice, you will find it easier to shift into this mode of attention whenever you wish. Even though the stress of pain or anxiety is very compelling, the more you practice bringing to it your full attention, the more skilled you become. When you become able to include this awareness in all your everyday interactions, you will notice that your life takes on a more wholehearted quality, as though you had more of yourself available for each thing that you do.

CONCENTRATION PRACTICE: DEVELOPING
THE "COMING-BACK" MUSCLE

One form of meditation practice is to focus your attention on just one thing, like your breath, carefully counting your inhalations and exhalations and noticing the pauses in between. Focusing on anything to the exclusion of everything else is called a concentration practice. You are developing your ability to focus all your attention on one particular thing and let everything else, no matter how potentially riveting, drop away. When you are doing a concentration practice, you not only notice when your attention is steadily focused on the object you have chosen, but you also notice when it wanders away. If you are new to meditation, you will probably be amazed at how often your mind wanders away from the object on which you have chosen to concentrate. This wandering quality is a basic propensity of the mind. I call it "puppy-mind," a tendency to run about and sniff everything.

It doesn't matter how many times your mind wanders away, perhaps thousands in a single half-hour meditation session. What's important is that you notice that your mind has wandered, and specifically where it has wandered to, then you gently disengage from that diversion and guide your attention back to your chosen focus, whatever that is. I think of concentration practice as developing the "coming-back" muscle. The more times your mind wanders away, the more opportunities you have to develop your ability to refocus your attention, to strengthen your coming-back muscle. Concentration meditation practice is not a matter of ruthlessly eliminating the random thoughts that tug at your attention; it is a matter of patiently and kindly, ideally without self-criticism or irritation, abandoning the side roads and turning your attention back to the object of your concentration. The following is a good practice to build up your coming-back muscle.

Wandering Mind Meditation

1. Arrange yourself in a position that is both stable and comfortable. (For detailed instructions concerning meditation

posture, see the "Instruction in Posture" section later in the chapter.)

2. Settle yourself and begin to notice your breath, specifically the inhalations and exhalations.
3. Without changing the rhythm or pace of your breath, begin to count the inhalations and exhalations from one to ten. An inhalation and an exhalation count as a pair. That is, the first time you breathe in, you say "one" in your mind; when you breathe out, you say "one" again. The next inhalation is "two"; the next exhalation is "two."
4. When you get to "ten," start over again, so that you are counting a continuous series of one to ten. Continue this throughout your period of meditation—say, for twenty to thirty minutes.

Whenever your attention leaves your counting, note specifically where it goes—for example, to what you have to do after this period of meditation, to a fantasy of what you'd rather be doing, to thoughts of irritation or agitation, to sleepiness, to a work project, whatever. It doesn't matter where it goes; what's important is that you gently return it to your breath and your counting. The counting is to help you notice that your attention has strayed. What may be especially interesting to you is where it goes. You may notice obsessive patterns and habits of mind you weren't aware of before starting this practice. No matter how many times you lose track of your counting, note where your attention goes, over and over again, and then gently bring it back to your counting. The Wandering Mind exercise both develops your coming-back muscle and reveals your own particular habits of mind, the favorite places you revisit again and again.

Obstacles to Concentration (Coursing with the Demons)

What is most difficult about meditation practice in general, and concentration practice in particular, is that you often have thoughts and feelings you would rather not have. In the normal course of your daily life, you tend to conveniently "overlook" thoughts and feelings that make you uncomfortable, to turn away from what makes you cringe. During a period of meditation, however, there they are, and you have nothing to do but notice them. Such discomfort can be very discouraging; thus, it is important to learn to observe what you think and feel without judging or criticizing your thoughts and feelings. This is called "bare recognition." Not only that, if you are to discover the compulsions, antipathies, and quirks of personality that intensify your suffering, you need to observe them with some dispassion. In fact, your relentless criticism of yourself could become an important part of your meditation practice: noticing whenever critical thoughts arise, how long it takes them to pass away of their own accord, and what kind of thoughts precede and follow them. Critical thoughts are just more grist for the meditation mill: simply observe that you tend to make judgments about your thoughts and feelings, and after you notice that you do this, you can move on to other thoughts and feelings.

Shunryu Suzuki-roshi, the founder of the San Francisco Zen Center, used to speak of our problems in meditation as the "weeds of enlightenment," which we pull up and use as compost to nourish our self-exploration. Weeds and flowers together are the seeds of our intention to become aware of all the aspects of our lives, be they dandelions or roses.

Halloween Ritual for Our Demons

At Zen Center in San Francisco, we hold an elaborate Halloween ritual. First of all, it's fun to come to the ceremony in costume, the way the kids do. Most of us dress up as a demon or a witch— something that acknowledges the shadow side of ourselves, which we honor in the ceremony. We set up an altar full of candles and fruit and candy and call forth the hungry ghosts. Hungry ghosts are beings described in Buddhist psychology whose bellies are enormous but whose mouths are tiny pinholes, so they can never eat enough to satisfy their voracious need. Thus, they roam desperately hungry and perpetually unsatisfied, like their human counterparts who find it impossible to be happy with what they have, always comparing it to their fantasy of what they should have or once had. At Halloween, all the bounty of harvesttime that we've put on the altar we offer to these roving, miserable spirits of craving.

We chant the "Gate of Sweet Dew" to the hungry ghosts and any random demons who might be present. Part of the "Gate of Sweet Dew" goes:

> We invite all deceased ancestors, the spirits of mountains, rivers and earth, and all the demons of untamed lands to come and assemble here. Now with compassion and empathy, we offer each of you food. We sincerely hope that each and every one of you will receive our offering, turn it over, and pass it on to all . . . sentient beings throughout the realm of vast emptiness. May you and all sentient beings together be fully satisfied. Again we hope your bodies will be conveyed by these offerings and mantras so that you may let go of all suffering, attain liberation, be born in heaven, receive joy, and play freely in the pure lands of the ten directions.

When the North Peninsula Sangha, which is a much smaller group than the San Francisco Zen Center, meets for Halloween, we step up to the altar individually in turn. After lighting a stick of incense, each of us calls forth our own personal demons by name. Last year, I called forth my self-indulgence and my arrogance. Other people called on selfishness, laziness, fear, lack of consideration for others. After calling forth our personal demons, each of us promises to protect and comfort the demons who answer our call to join us. We invite them to eat and chant with us in the safe place we are creating together. People report being very moved at this ceremony, saying it gives them a different perspective on the personal character traits they always find so annoying and wish would go away.

I mention this ceremony because I think it represents a very accepting and compassionate attitude toward our so-called flaws that is very useful in our meditation practice. We can sit and become aware of our demons and ghosts, our old habit patterns, and invite them to join us in our meditation in hopes that they will be fed and put at ease, so that they may cease to roam the earth in desperation. Once settled peacefully beside us, they may give up to us their storehouse of energy and clarity that we have bound up in perceiving them as demons.

Referring to these mental annoyances as "demons" is very dramatic; it makes them quite clear to us, giving them personal characteristics. Actually, these mental states were first referred to as "demons" by Christian meditators in ancient times. Buddhists call them "hindrances," specific states of mind that interfere with clarity. Vipashyanā tradition considers the naming of these states to be "the first step in bringing them to a wakeful conscious attention." (See Jack Kornfield, *A Path with Heart.*) Buddha directed meditators to note "This is a mind filled with joy" and "This is a mind fueled with anger," acknowledging each state as it arose and passed away.

Whether you prefer to practice with "demons" or "hindrances," I think it is useful to recognize their presence and their continual arising and passing, not only during formal meditation periods but in your daily life, so that you have some perspective from which to view your critical, self-pitying, or obsessive mind. If you understand these states of mind as "demons" or "hindrances," it's easier to question the viewpoint they bring to your consciousness. After you come to have a pretty good idea of what your particular favorites are, you can choose one on which to concentrate for days or weeks, or you can notice several of them in a single period of meditation whenever they appear.

If you are new to meditation, I recommend that you spend the first couple of weeks developing breathing as your ground of being before you take on noticing your demons when they appear. Once you feel settled in your breathing and can return to it after discovering yourself riding out on a train of thought (that is, when you've built up the coming-back muscle a little), that might be a good time to begin the practice of noting or naming your individual demons. Perhaps you can start with one in particular and notice what bodily feelings or images accompany it and possibly what mind states precede and follow it.

The following list includes both traditional "demons" or "hindrances" and the ones most often remarked upon by meditators whom I know personally. If you have one or two of your own that aren't listed here, please don't hesitate to adapt the suggestions for practicing with other demons to your unique situation.

Desire. Many people are miserable because their mental lives are spent mostly in wanting, fantasizing, collecting objects or pleasant states of mind, then helplessly watching them pass away. Experiencing the pleasure right there in front of you, a relaxing massage or a delicious meal, or appreciating beautiful objects that you love, is not the problem. It's wanting what you don't have or grasping what you're afraid to lose that's the problem. If dwelling on the bliss that would be yours "if only," or on your particular paradise lost, is a mental habit for you, it is important to get to know the shadings of this thought pattern so intimately—what it feels like to have it and what events or feelings evoke it—that you can distinguish greed and want from the real pleasure that experiences and objects give you.

If your mind has this disposition, your meditation will be filled with fantasies of attaining intangibles (admiration, peace of mind, security) and acquiring tangibles (wealth, a new car, a vacation). If you find this series of chasing-afters tiresome, it behooves you to begin to investigate the thought patterns that enslave you in the realm of desire. There is no need to actually get rid of any desire. If you closely observe the way your mind plunges itself into craving, gradually developing the patience required to stay with the unpleasantness of the feeling until it passes, you should eventually be able to detect an opening in your craving large enough that you can experience desire without enslavement.

If you get so familiar with the feelings you experience when you view the steady parade of the things/experiences/self-esteem you covet, you may lapse enough in your hankering that you can occasionally turn your attention to what you already have and feel yourself pleased. Then your habit of greed will feel more like spotting an ice cream parlor next to the restaurant you're just leaving. You want a hot fudge sundae, but since you couldn't put another thing in your stomach, you don't want it, too. So you pass it up with a smile, thinking of how you love and appreciate everything there is in the world. This is a very different involvement with the objects of desire than the compulsive obsession of addiction.

Critical Mind. Many people are plagued with continual critical thoughts about themselves and everything around them. They can't enjoy a meal, a piece of music, another person's company, their own competence, without judgmental thoughts that strangle the life out of everything they perceive. Some may have internalized a parent's constant criticism as a child; others may have developed a highly refined aesthetic that they can't set aside at will, even when they would rather relax than judge—for instance, a food critic who can't enjoy a meal cooked by a friend who is merely an adequate cook. In meditation practice, this manifests as constant worry that you're not doing it right, you never could do anything right, the atmosphere is not conducive, and so on.

If you try to get rid of these judgments by thinking you shouldn't judge, then you're just making another judgment. Instead, try acknowledging the judgment as it arises. Allow it to come and go. Judgments are often a tape from childhood or from an encounter with another person's opinion that plays through the mind over and over again. It is helpful to notice how these thoughts feel in your body: their impact on your muscles, breath, any discomfort you usually have in sitting still. It could also be quite illuminating to count your judgments through the day and see how much of your conscious life is shaped by this constant perception of "wrong" and "not good enough." Notice what patterns of energy or tension reflect this mental state as well as your resistance to it.

When I was relatively new to meditation, I was so harshly critical of my own meditation practice that I was often very discouraged and sought reassurance from my teacher. I would wail to him, "Oh, I can't concentrate, I can't sit still, I can't follow my breath," on and on until one morning he said very firmly, "Don't criticize anything for a year! That means that when you turn the radio on in the car, don't turn to another station because you don't like the one that's on. When you're at a movie, just watch how it was made without thinking about what's wrong with it. When you eat a meal, just eat without thinking about how you've had better!" I left the room strongly determined to follow his suggestion.

The first thing that happened was, I ran into another Zen student in the hall and immediately thought, "God, why can't that woman wash her hair occasionally!" Whoops! Chagrined at my immediate lapse into "critical mind," I cut off the thought about her hair and vowed to be less critical. I went down the stairs into the street and noticed a grubby-looking, apparently homeless man gathering cans and bottles that had been dropped by the curb. Immediately I was flooded with judgments about him and his filth, the carelessness of people discarding trash, and the city government that allowed people to live in this condition. Horrified by my virtual torrent of judgments, I hurried upstairs to my apartment. There was my husband, snoring away into the dawn while I had been virtuously sitting in meditation and had even had an interview with my teacher. "What a slug!" leaped to mind before I could stay the judgment. I sat down unhappily on the bed and put my chin in my hands. I had always considered myself the least critical, most easygoing of women! Yet in the ten minutes that had barely passed since my teacher gave me this practice, I had had virtually none but critical thoughts!

You might take the trouble to note whether critical thoughts speak in your mind with any particular voice. I believed my critical mind when it told me I was incompetent and wayward, until I recognized the voice in my mind telling me that as my father's. I had to laugh then because when I was a teenager, I consciously thought my dad was a total idiot and never listened to anything he said. I apparently still had that opinion of his advice, even though I had internalized the content and come to believe it, because when I recognized his scolding voice as the source of my critical thoughts about myself and my future, I was instantly relieved of them.

Some people suffer tremendously from their sense that life has ultimately been disappointing, but they don't realize that they themselves poison every experience by criticizing it to death. They just think the whole world is substandard, that they alone have been cursed or blessed with the proper ideals from which to judge. One afternoon, I led workshop participants in a brief meditation on sound. I instructed them to allow various sounds to arise and subside in their consciousness, some appearing alone and some overlapping. We were nearly a hundred people in a large room next to a busy street. Very few of them had ever done such a meditation before. When I asked for comments afterward, several people remarked that it had been extremely relaxing, even blissful, to concentrate on simple sounds as a break from their usual insistent thought patterns. After several remarks along this line, I asked if anyone had had a hard time. One woman immediately raised her hand. "What was hard?" I asked her. "Well, it was really hard to concentrate with that noisy ventilation system in here, people not sitting still in their chairs, and that terrible traffic outside," she said. "I couldn't hear anything! This is really a poor room to meditate in."

She had such a strong idea of which sounds she would like to hear and which ones were annoying, I suggested that a long-term meditation practice that might be helpful to her would be to observe her critical thoughts. Clearly thunderstruck, she demanded sharply, "What do you mean?" I admit I was a little intimidated by such a strong reaction to my suggestion. "I mean," I began, "that since you used the words *noisy* and *terrible* to describe the sounds you heard, maybe you were too preoccupied with judging the sounds rather than listening to them." She was stunned into silence. I felt uncomfortable, concerned that I had spoken too directly in front of so many people. I went on to take other questions but continued to feel bad about what I perceived as laying an unwanted trip on someone.

She came up to me at the break, about an hour later. Bracing myself for the worst, I hoped to disarm her by apologizing, but she spoke first. "Thank you," she said. I couldn't believe my ears or the warm expression on her face. "Thank you," she repeated.

"I've gone to meditation workshops before, but nobody has ever suggested I look at what kind of thoughts I have. I started doing what you suggested immediately, and you were right. I never simply hear anything. I'm always laying a trip on it. In just this afternoon, I see what the others were talking about when they said they felt relieved from their usual thoughts. It's such a relief just to hear." She hugged me. I looked into her face. She looked truly relaxed and very beautiful.

Sleepiness. In the long hotel corridor of our minds, the door to sleep is right next to the door to meditative awareness. That's because we're used to falling asleep when we feel relaxed or still. The mind in meditation, on the other hand, is both relaxed and alert. We feel at ease and calm, but instead of falling asleep we are much more aware than usual, attuned to any sensory stimulation or idea that arises. It takes some practice to be able to distinguish between the relaxation that is heightened awareness and the relaxation that leads to drowsiness and then be able to choose to be alert right in the middle of the drowsiness.

It might take some time to break the mind's association of sleep with relaxation. This will take patience and determination. When we are relaxed and alert, there is a lightness to our bodies, a liveliness about our attention. We are ready for anything. In contrast, sleepiness in meditation arises as fuzziness, tiredness, lack of vitality. The body feels heavy, unable to hold a posture; the eyes close against our will, without our notice. We don't know we have been asleep until we are startled awake. Nothing seems more important than indulging this weariness. We can't remember why in the world we would want to try to stay awake instead of just going to sleep.

The difficulty with sleepiness in meditation is this very fogginess and the disappearance of our intention to concentrate. In order to overcome this demon, we have to focus on it at the very moment when we are most unfocused. It helps to sit up straight, take deep breaths, and focus the mind on something specific, like this very breath, very much like grabbing onto a passing lifeboat if we are drowning. Anything we can hang onto or affix our attention to will help. It can be especially useful to focus on the mental and physical elements of our sleepiness itself. Sleepiness is a hard demon to penetrate; it washes over us with such alluring sweetness. But we have spent so much of our lives unconscious and unaware of our living, both awake and asleep, it behooves us to shake off our covers and wake up!

Compulsive Mind, Restlessness. This hindrance—experienced as agitation, nervousness, anxiety, and worry—is known in Buddhism as Pacing Tiger meditation. It is hell to sit there and be in your body, your particular mind, this very room. You'd rather do anything else. In this case, the way out is definitely in. Become the world's expert at knowing every exact, excruciating little detail about what agitation is: the tension, the boredom, the physical restlessness, the energy, the resistance, the far-flung thoughts, the sheer desperation. If you decide to observe everything about this state of mind, you penetrate it; it actually becomes absorbing!

What's required here is that you open yourself, surrender yourself to the restlessness, without buying into its seductions: what you have to do next, the deadline at the end of the week, how you're wasting your time, how much your body wants to move. Just experience it without believing the line with which it's trying to seduce you: planning the party for your child's birthday next May, making the grocery list now because it will save you a few minutes after meditation. Simply allow these thoughts to move through without sticking. Even though compulsive planning may be a fairly ingrained habit of mind, if you get familiar with its elements, you'll be able to see how transitory and insubstantial this state is. Which is more important—the grocery list or your ease of mind?

Your meditation periods aren't the only times for you to conquer this most insidious of mental habits, this thief of your days, this ravisher of the moments of your life! Learn through your growing familiarity with the attributes of this habit to confine your planning, your listing, your figuring out logistics to a time you set aside for them. If they wake you up in the middle of the night, give them ten minutes, then relax into your breathing and go back to sleep. If they creep into your lovemaking, your spectacular sunset, firmly tell them to wait their turn—and then give them a turn. Sit down with a cup of tea and figure it all out.

When I was going through a terrible crisis in my life, I worried so much all the time, I realized I was ruining my whole life with this one concern. So I set aside worry time each day to let my mind run rampant with anxiety, hoping thereby to free the rest of the time. As it turned out, it wasn't so much the worry time itself that was so useful; it was the ability to say to my compulsive mind whenever the worry arose that it had to leave me alone now—I would indulge it later. This is how you treat a clamoring child: with respect and promises of your company later. This is taking seriously the habits of our mind so that we can begin to free ourselves.

A friend of mine took three extensions on his income tax. For a good four months, I heard him natter and complain about how when he finally sat down and did the forms, it would be a hellish job. At the movies, over dinner, he would relax, and the relaxation itself would trigger the anxiety-producing topic: his undone income taxes! How could he relax when they were still out there, waiting for his attention! Finally he set aside a weekend to do them. He nearly faltered when the weekend arrived and the weather was gorgeous, but no, he was going to do the taxes no matter what. He brought all the forms to his desk. He gathered sharpened pencils, receipts, a calculator. He resolutely closed the curtains. He sat down to work. He was done in an hour and a half. His projected weekend in hell ended at noon on Saturday! He phoned me, half-mad with relief and self-disgust. "I can't believe it!" he cried. "All those moments of my life wasted worrying about doing the income taxes! I swear I will never again waste my life thinking about something I have to do until I sit down and do it!" Do you think that will be true?

Doubting Mind. I have a good friend with whom I traveled to Europe who inadvertently gave me a front-row seat to watch "doubting mind" in action. Every morning, she laid out all her clothes on the bed and chose an outfit to wear. So far, so good. But immediately after the choice was made, she became agitated, uncomfortable. "Do you think I should wear the dress instead of the pants?" she would appeal to me. At first, naively hoping to be of help, I would say, "The dress." Then she would argue with me. "No, I think the pants would be better; it might get chilly." Wherever she came down—on her outfit, the wine purchase, the cheese preference, the castle tour instead of the art museum—she immediately leaped into doubting mind, questioning the choice she had just made.

Seeing this pattern she exhibited with trivial things, I remembered her agony over the years with decisions about past boyfriends, whether they were good for her or had enough affection for her. In recent years, she has been enjoying a solid relationship with a remarkable man, but she is continually questioning whether the relationship should continue in the face of its problems: he is a single parent; he doesn't like to go dancing; they live forty minutes apart. Frequently by his words or actions, he is able to convince her that he loves her deeply, but she is always wondering, Does this or that behavior or comment mean that he doesn't love me? Do my dogs love him enough? Ironically, it's precisely because she has committed herself to him in her heart that she has these constant doubts. Otherwise, she would appear to be the strong, faithful person she actually is. It is the commitment itself that stirs doubting mind.

My husband also has the habit of doubting mind. He never met an expert at anything whose opinion he trusted. When a repairman inspected our roof and gave an estimate, what I heard the repairman say was that the damage (and thus the expense) was less than we had expected. What my husband heard was that we were going to be swindled and bankrupted. Before we bought this house, my husband was the driving force behind its purchase. Since we bought it, he has been driving himself crazy with doubts about our decision.

What it takes to ease the bondage of doubting mind is enough understanding of it to let it arise and pass out of the mind without sticking. Like compulsive mind, doubting mind only has power if you believe its story. What if my life is ruined? What if I'm being deceived? Am I being made a victim here? These thoughts are like children pulling at your skirts while you're trying to walk. If you can allow yourself some aloofness while being assailed by them, because you have become so familiar with their pattern, you're as good as free of them. Actually, when harnessed and no longer acting as an energy-sucking demon, doubting mind can gather itself into a force for penetrating the surface of our lives and deepening our experience of reality. It can be the "Show me!" that cuts through facile answers or conventional wisdom. When you doubt experts, then you must rely on your own experience. The clarity about what is ultimately important is developed through coming to know doubting mind intimately and cultivating the patience to let it come and go, an old friend whose opinions are strong but a little erratic.

༜

WHEN WE BECOME SKILLFUL at noticing our habits of mind and letting them come and go without disturbing us, we realize that each state of mind, including strong emotions, only lasts for seconds before being replaced by another one. Anger turns to sadness, which turns to melancholy, which turns to comfort, which turns to relaxation, which turns to enjoyment, and so on. We come to appreciate that the underlying nature of puppy-mind is actually a ceaseless, uninterrupted flow of thoughts and feelings. When we understand this truth, we can choose to settle into the awareness of each thought or feeling as it arises and passes. In this way, we cultivate some freedom from the frantic imbalance created by each one.

Demon Meditation

Choose one of your demons and be aware of it, in both your formal meditation periods and your daily life, for a whole week without trying to change it or get away from it. What happens when you stay there?

BASIC AWARENESS

Concentration practices are very helpful in developing the ability to focus the attention and to observe the flitting about of puppy-mind, but meditation that does not have an object of focus more specific than whatever is before us is more like the quality of our attention in everyday life. In our normal day-to-day lives, our attention is drawn from one thing to another all day long: the reassuring sound of a car braking as we step from the curb, the expression on a coworker's face as we outline a project, the logistics of a weekend trip that we're planning, fantasies of wealth and physical ease, the surge of desire when an attractive person smiles, hunger pangs just before lunch, and so on. Actually, we are fortunate indeed if all these stimuli successfully draw our notice because we are just as likely to spend much of the day preoccupied with mental habits that are powerful enough to prevent us from being aware of the myriad events all around us. This is when our lives take on a dampened, incomplete quality. If we actually notice this dissatisfaction, we may feel restless, yearning for more "intensity" or "meaning" in our lives.

The meditation practice that develops the ability to pay attention to everything at once is called *shikan taza* (Japanese for "just sitting"). "Just sitting" means we don't do anything extra during our meditation, like concentrate on a particular object or bring our minds back to a particular focus or even tell ourselves that now we are meditating. We just are quiet and still enough that we can observe how our minds behave, whether they are dull and distracted, whether they pay attention to breathing, whether they are alert and receptive, whether they work out the details of a project. We don't do anything to change what is actually going on. In this context, our compulsive thinking and critical judgments are not "demons," to be recognized and abandoned for our breath practice; rather, they are the show itself. Because shikan taza demands consistent awareness, many people may find it a more difficult practice than simply concentrating on one object, but it is also a radically enlivening practice.

Shikan Taza

1. Sit comfortably in a position that is both stable and relaxed. (For a detailed discussion of meditation posture, see the "Instruction in Posture" section later in the chapter.)

2. Specifically notice your breathing and your body sensations as you settle into your comfortable but alert posture. Notice your inhalations, your exhalations, and the pauses in between. Following the breath is the entryway to shikan taza.

3. After you feel settled into your breathing and posture, open out your focus a little and begin to take in everything there is: the sensations and gurgles of your internal physical world, the stimulation of the external world as it comes in through your senses, the thoughts that arise spontaneously to your consciousness and then pass, and the emotional feelings that color your awareness.

   You may be able to take in all these things in your immediate environment for a decent period of time before you veer off on a string of thoughts that exclude everything else you have been aware of. This is because, if you're like most people, thinking thoughts is your dominant mode of consciousness. One thought usually leads to another and then another and then another until you notice you are thinking thoughts to the exclusion of everything else. At that point, you might open out your focus again to include your whole world. Or you might choose to continue your train of thought, only now you are aware that you have been thinking.

Shikan taza is like being at the theater watching a live play, only the actors are your thoughts and feelings. Notice how you like to spend your mental time, the fantasies and patterns that occur repeatedly, and how you actually prefer languishing in them to being aware of them as merely one aspect of the present moment. Note how this differs from day to day, what mood or background feeling you bring to your meditation. This will give you an idea of your general disposition and how it varies over time.

The content of shikan taza meditation can be anything. What's important in this meditation is the attitude, the open awareness of anything that appears. No matter what is manifesting in your mind, you are clearly aware, open to revelation. Even if you are very upset, angry at yourself for not being calm during your period of meditation, in the midst of that you're clearly aware of what is happening—your being upset and disappointed. This awareness is a state of mind beyond words. You don't have to stop the upset. Some part of you that is not upset and angry is being refined right in the midst of your anger and upset. In the words of twelfth-century Zen master Dogen, you're like a "tiger when she enters the mountains" or the "dragon when he gains the water." Shikan taza is not about self-improvement, making your mind state better or more acceptable. It's about developing a part of you that yearns to be alive, to discover a radiant clarity beyond words and thought.

INSTRUCTION IN POSTURE

All meditation postures share two very important points: (1) the stability of the lower body and (2) the straightness of the spine. The feeling of stability in the lower body makes it possible for us to sit through turmoil and fear; the straight spine gives the body a feeling of lightness and support that keeps us alert. Of course, many of us have physical difficulties that prevent us from assuming the traditional meditation postures, so if it is impossible for us to straighten our spines completely for whatever reason, we must work with what we have. (See the "Alternative Postures" subsection later in the chapter.)

Classic Meditation Postures

The classic meditation postures that have come down through the ages to us are variants on cross-legged sitting:

Cross-Legged Sitting. This posture usually requires at least two different cushions: a large, square one that serves as an area rug for your sitting and supports your whole body, especially your knees, which will probably rest directly upon it, and a smaller firm, thick, round cushion (called a zafu) to lift and support your rear end. How thick your zafu should be depends on the flexibility of your knees and spine. The less angle your knees will allow, the thicker your zafu should be. What's important is that your rear end be higher than your knees, but the weight distribution between them should be almost even. If your knees are tight enough that they won't rest on the large, square cushion once you are on your zafu, put little pillows or towels underneath your knees to support them. Don't let them hang in the air. This not only creates tension in your legs and back, but it drastically reduces the stability you feel in this posture.

You may have to experiment with different zafus and support cushions for some time before you get just the right combination. I also advise a few minutes of stretching exercises before sitting in meditation so that you can gradually lengthen your front and back thigh muscles to accommodate your sitting posture more easily. A variety of excellent exercises can be found in yoga books or on the Internet; choose the best ones for your particular body. Don't be impatient about the tightness of your body, or you'll tear some tissue and be out of commission for a while. Just assume you'll be doing this activity for an indefinite time into the future and allow your pelvis and thighs to stretch out at their own pace.

Once you have determined the optimum placement of the cushions to support your rear end and knees, turn your attention to the placement of your arms and hands. Your arms should be slightly away from your body rather than held closely to your sides. The rule of thumb is a distance large enough so that you could be holding an egg in each armpit. Bring your hands together at the tops of your thighs. This classic mudra, or way of holding your hands, is to place the back of your right hand on the very top of your right thigh with the palm open and the fingers together. Place the back of your left hand in the palm of your right hand so that the fingers of the left hand completely cover the fingers of the right hand, and the left fingertips meet the pads of the right hand where the bottoms of the fingers start (the metacarpals).

This leaves your thumbs in the air, facing each other. Just barely touch the tips of the thumbs together, so that your hands and thumbs form an oval that surrounds your navel. The advantage of this mudra is that when, in meditation, you notice your thumbs jammed together, you realize you are too tense, probably thinking compulsive thoughts or following a train of thought very closely. When you notice that your thumbs have fallen away from each other, you realize you are sleepy or daydreaming. It takes some attention to keep the thumbs barely touching—a mindfulness practice within an awareness practice.

If you find this mudra too difficult for physical reasons, just place your hands in any comfortable but conscious position: palms down on your thighs, palms up on your thighs, intertwined and resting in your lap, or loosely held together in your lap. I have designed a mudra especially for my arthritic hands: my hands rest palms down in my lap with my thumbs and first fingers of both hands forming a diamond with the rest of the fingers relaxed. The point is, your hands and arms should add to the stable feeling of your overall posture without being jammed against your sides. A mudra also adds a locus of awareness.

With your lower body stable and your hands placed comfortably, bring your attention to your head. Tuck in your chin so that the crown of your head (this is not the very top of your head; it is more toward the top back of your head) extends toward the sky. In fact, when you feel yourself unbalanced or slumping during meditation, correct from the crown, stretching your spine by extending the crown of your head toward the sky rather than tensing your lower back muscles. Not only does extending your crown to the sky align your whole upper body, it also relieves the pressure that can be put on the disks in your lower back when you correct your posture by arching your back. Your upper teeth should rest lightly on your lower teeth, with the same ease as your thumbs touch in the classic mudra.

Because you are in the process of permeating your whole life with your meditation, rather than retiring to a private world of ethereal mental realms, you keep your eyes open during meditation. Drop your gaze to the floor a few feet beyond your knees. Relax your gaze enough so that your eyes are slightly unfocused. You're not actively looking at anything; your visual world is just another aspect of your meditation.

In your sitting, it is advisable to maintain a dynamic tension between comfort and alertness. You want to be comfortable enough that your attention is not continually pulled to any discomfort, which might lead to your constantly readjusting your position. Yet you don't want to feel so at ease that you fall asleep or lose your edge, the ability to make the great effort that it takes to maintain your awareness of everything within and around you. The ideal posture is relaxed and comfortable but contains elements of tension: the placement of your hands, your jaw, your knees, the maintenance of a straight spine. A formal mudra requires monitoring, pulling your attention out of a fantasy to notice that your thumbs are jammed against each other rather than just touching. If you place your upper teeth gently upon your lower teeth, you may notice when your jaw goes slack that you have fallen asleep or stopped receiving information from your senses in favor of some internal dialogue. It is this kind of relaxed but alert attention that transforms the automatic quality of a routine life into a vibrant awareness that imbues any daily activity with the experience of breath, body, thought, and feeling.

Here are some variants on the cross-legged posture:

Full Lotus. The tops of both feet are placed on the tops of the opposite thighs. This is the maximally stable posture. Your back virtually aligns itself, and there is very little tension in your neck and shoulders. If you can get into this posture, that's great, since you won't have to work much at stability and alignment.

Half Lotus. The top of one foot is placed on the top of the opposite thigh. If you're like most people, you'll find you have a side preference, which could lead to your hips and back getting unbalanced fairly early in your meditation practice. Because it is hard on your back to continue to fuel this imbalance, it is best to alternate your feet in half lotus. I advise exercises to equalize the two sides of your body and to stretch out the tighter side. Again, refer to a yoga book or exercises on the Internet for sitting meditation.

Burmese Style. This is cross-legged sitting with the legs merely folded alongside each other on the square cushion in front of you, without your feet pulled up onto the thighs.

Seiza. The knees are bent under you, and you sit on your lower legs and feet. You can put either a zafu or a smaller cushion between your rear end and your heels, or you can purchase a small bench for this purpose called a seiza bench. Seiza benches may be purchased through the San Francisco Zen Center Bookstore (415-863-3136). The rest of the instructions for hands, head, and eyes are the same as for the cross-legged postures.

Alternative Postures

Because so many people have physical problems that interfere with or prevent their taking traditional cross-legged sitting postures in meditation, I have developed alternative sitting, standing, walking, and lying postures that may be of use to you. I first realized there was a need for such alternatives while teaching a meditation class at the Recreational Center for the Handicapped in San Francisco because a few elderly and disabled people had asked me to do so. I had already been teaching a movement class in the pool every week for people in pain, and the unspoken basis of that class was meditation. I led participants in slow loosening and stretching movements, always emphasizing awareness of body sensation (the feeling against the skin of our bathing suits and the ripple of water as we moved) and sensory input (the smell of the chlorine, the sound of the pool pump, the sight of all of us moving together). Although I never mentioned the word *meditation,* a few of the students (mostly women in their sixties and seventies with joint and back problems) caught on. They arranged for a room at the center and asked me to instruct them in formal meditation on dry land.

We used the available conference chairs and gathered pillows to adjust the chairs to our individual body parts. After an initial guided meditation through the body, I taught them Wandering Mind (presented earlier in the chapter) and eventually shikan taza. After our group had met four or five times, one of the most disabled women came up to me after class and put her hand on my arm. "All these years, I've wanted to meditate," she told me with tears in her eyes, "but since I couldn't sit cross-legged, I thought I never could in this lifetime." How poignant it was to hear this! Having already begun my meditation practice before my joints got so stiff, I never thought twice about continuing when I could no longer sit cross-legged. I just sat in other ways. But when she said that to me, I realized how people who had not been sitting in meditation before their difficulty might assume that that activity was now closed to them forever. Right then, I decided to invent as many alternative postures as I could think of, and I approached Vicki Austin, a Zen priest and yoga teacher, to help me. Here are some of the variations we came up with, along with more classical alternatives:

Sitting in a Chair. This is probably the most complicated meditation posture because, chairs being what they are, it's difficult to find one that suits your particular body. Pillows will be needed to adjust you to whatever chair you have available. What's important here are the same things that are important in cross-legged sitting: the stability of the lower body and the alignment of the spine. They're just harder to achieve in a chair. If you have short legs, you may need a cushion under your feet for your lower body to feel stable and solidly placed. If your feet fall asleep during your meditation period, it might be because your knees are enough lower than your rear end that the edge of the chair seat is cutting off your circulation. In this case, you need a pillow to elevate your knees to the level of your hips. On the other hand, if you are too tall for your chair, you may need a firm cushion under your rear end so that both of your feet, heel and toe, are firmly planted on the floor.

Once your feet are planted, you can see to your back. To get my feet planted firmly on the floor, I need to sit on the edge of a chair, which often leaves a huge gap between my back and the back of the chair. If my back tires, I put a very thick pillow between my lower back and the back of the chair to fill in the gap. If your back is not straight, a couple of very distracting things will happen: either you will get sleepy, or your shoulders and neck will ache afterward from the tension of holding up your upper body. You need to adjust pillows behind you so that your back is straight enough that you feel no tension in your shoulders, neck, or upper back from supporting your body. You may feel other tension, perhaps chronic tension, in those areas, but it shouldn't be because you haven't aligned your spine in a way that encourages your stable lower body to support your upper body.

You can tuck in your chin, lower your eyes, and arrange your hands as indicated for the cross-legged postures in the preceding subsection.

Walking Meditation. Walking meditation consists of walking slowly in a contained way so as to promote awareness of the body and breath while taking steps. Start by standing with your feet far enough apart that one is under each breast. Your hands can take one of many contained positions: clasped together at your belly or behind you, hanging at your sides, or in the traditional mudra of elbows bent, left hand in a fist, right hand around the left fist with the right thumb on top of the left thumb.

When you begin walking, deliberately place your foot on the floor so that you are conscious of the contact. Some people plant their toes first before their heels, adding another dimension of awareness. I plant my heel first because the calves of my legs are tight and I like to use every walking opportunity to gently stretch them. You can do either. Walk slowly enough that you are aware of the sensations of your muscles as you shift from one leg to the other.

Some people come to love walking meditation and do it frequently, not only formally during a regular meditation period but informally, whenever they are walking someplace. If you are a beginner, though, it is important to realize that walking meditation is different from the goal-directed walking you usually do to get somewhere. When you do walking meditation, the mind is focused on the experience of walking. You allow your mind to follow each step. It is of course possible to adapt your everyday walking to walking meditation even when you are walking to someplace, but when doing so you should remember to notice the minutiae of your bodily feelings and sensations as well as noting your distance from your destination. Chapter 11 contains additional suggestions for walking meditation.

Pacing. Pacing is fast walking meditation, done at a speed much closer to normal walking. For people with particular back problems like sciatica or herniated disk, speeding up the walking offers the advantage of easing back pain. Faster walking tends to stretch the vertebrae (as long as it is done with a pelvis loose enough that it is drawn forward from the lower back with each step), whereas very slow walking extends the amount of time that there is pressure on the lower back from one leg being behind the body. Even though the pace is a bit faster, the containment and awareness exemplified by walking meditation should be maintained.

Rather than pacing open-endedly, choose a specific area, like the perimeter of a room or up and down a path or hallway, and keep going over it again and again. If you are in a meditation hall with other people, you may want to pace a distance from them in a part of the hall that can be yours or even outside in the entry area. Some meditation halls have walkways around them for walking meditation, which would work very well for pacing during formal periods. In the pacing posture, the hands may be placed in one of the positions suggested for walking meditation. The challenge in this posture may be to maintain your awareness of your individual steps during such a familiar and habitual activity.

Standing. Place your whole body against a straight wall with several points of contact: the back of your head, your heels, and as much of your spine, including your lower spine, as possible. This demands that you tuck your pelvis forward in order to contact the wall with your lower spine. This is the tension in this posture; you have to maintain your pelvic tuck or restore it when it relaxes. Maintaining this posture demands a great deal of concentration, which is one of its advantages. It might be an antidote to chronic sleepiness.

Lying on the Back. Lying on the back is a great posture for those of us with joint problems and/or muscle tension because the body weight is distributed over the whole spine. The problem with lying down during meditation has always been that we inevitably fall asleep. We are just too used to going to sleep when we lie down. Even though we may be determined to keep our eyes open and our minds alert, the habit and comfort are just too much to overcome. In this situation, the balance between comfort and the tension that promotes alertness is so seriously tilted toward ease that alertness is compromised. So Vicki and I have introduced some tension into the posture to overcome the obstacle of too little tension in the body.

Lie on your back with your knees bent and lightly touching each other, your feet firmly on the floor, and the insides of your feet lightly touching each other. The tension in this posture is just this—keeping the knees and feet together. If you start to drift, the knees will part. Put a firm cushion (a zafu is ideal) on your chest. With your elbows on the floor for support, place your hands across from each other on the cushion so as to form some personal mudra, meaning that your hands are consciously and symmetrically arranged on the cushion rather than resting there haphazardly. You will also notice the tendency of the cushion on your chest to rise and fall with your breath. Very cool. Feel free to place a small pillow (not one so soft it would encourage dozing) under your head or neck if you need support for either one. Your eyes should remain open.

Lying on the Side. Lie on your side (either side) with your legs as straight as you can make them and the top leg completely on top of, and supported by, the bottom leg. This, you will notice, is a hard posture to maintain without alertness; if you fall asleep, you will topple over. This is the tension that keeps you awake in this posture. The arm underneath can be bent under you or lie out straight on the floor underneath or in front of you. If this is uncomfortable, put a pillow between your arm and your head. The arm on top should be lying straight along the body with your hand ending up near your hip. Keep your eyes open.

Throughout all these alternative postures for meditation, the essence of the traditional meditation postures is retained: the stability of the lower body, the alignment of the spine, the focus of the mind, and the understanding that whatever waves our mind and body produce during our meditation period, they are not different from or separate from the big, wide, incomprehensible ocean itself.

Regularity of Practice

Many people sit down to meditate every day for thirty to forty minutes. Personally, I think it best to meditate formally five or six days a week because I notice some difference when I resume meditating after a day off; maybe it's just being glad to be back. Less than thirty minutes might be too short a period because it takes a while to settle. You might become discouraged with your practice if you get up day after day before you've given yourself a chance to settle, to relax into your posture, to notice your state of mind.

If you find it difficult to set aside time during a special project at work, a crisis in your life, or a period of travel, be patient and just keep trying. If you're like many people I know, you will discover deep pools of ingenuity you didn't know you had. You'll start counting your breaths in elevators, on airplanes, in taxis. You'll get up earlier in the morning. You'll plop down on the zafu while your children are getting ready for bed and pop up again when it's time to read them a story. You'll do walking meditation while your coffee is brewing or shikan taza while your dinner is cooking. You only have to abandon the idea that medi-

tation is something special that must be approached in a particular state of mind.

PHYSICAL PAIN DURING FORMAL MEDITATION PERIODS

If you have a lot of physical pain during your meditation periods,
it may be because you are tense or your body doesn't like to be
in one position or your restlessness and resistance take a physical
path. There are a couple of things you can do about this pain,
both of which involve treating your pain with great respect:

1. *Use your breath to expand the spaces in your body, thereby releasing
some tension.* Even though you are still, you are not motionless. If
you find that instead of becoming looser or more relaxed, you
become stiffer, tenser, and more ossified while sitting still, you
can use your breath to keep your meditation dynamic. Unrestricted breathing creates a natural rhythm for your body's functions,
and it can be a great comfort for you if you hand yourself over to
your breath in meditation. By that, I mean just let your breath
take over. Make it your primary focus. Let it expand you wherever
it will go.

Stiff, contracted people desperately need the sense of ease and
coordination that breath can lend to their sense of their bodies.
People in pain yearn for the spaciousness that breath creates
around everything: body parts, movements, thoughts, and events.
If you focus on your breath for even a few minutes in a row, you'll
glimpse an alternate reality that is compelling in its potential to
transform the way you currently endure your pain. When I become very concentrated on my breath, fully settling into its
rhythm of inhalation, pause, exhalation, pause, over and over
again, I feel as if I am in a wind tunnel or a hurricane, so extraordinarily aware am I of the sound and the movement breath
causes in my body.

2. *Adjust your position so as to ease the pain.* In order to develop
stability during formal meditation, it's usual not to move for the

entire period you've set yourself, refusing to be disturbed by an itch or a scratch, or a thought that arises in the mind for an instant. If you don't act on it, it passes quickly. I think it's best to sit through this kind of experience. When I first started sitting formal meditation, I sat daily in a very hot climate out in the woods. All kinds of insects would land on me: in my hair, on my arms, even on my nose or cheeks. Bees would walk along my legs, investigating the sweat behind my knees. Yuck. I hated it. At first, I would bat them away, but I soon realized that unless I ignored them, I would be spending all my meditation time shooing them. So I settled down and let them all do what they would. The results were such an encouragement to a new meditator! With itches unscratched and bugs crawling on me constantly, I felt like a mountain!

So it's quite desirable to sit still through discomfort in meditation, but it's different with pain. Pain often becomes gradually more insistent until it takes over your consciousness and you become upset and agitated. You might choose to sit through this kind of pain just to watch your mind deal with it. That's certainly acceptable, even laudable. I also think, however, that you might consider adjusting your posture to relieve the pain, especially if you find it so discouraging that you consider stopping your meditation practice. You can stretch out for a moment and resume your posture, or you can change to a new posture. When adjusting your posture to accommodate pain, it is important to move with the same deliberateness, the same concentration, the same observation of your feelings that you practice when you sit still. Feel how the pain is relieved. Notice the thoughts that accompany this relief. Notice what it takes to settle down again. And notice the thoughts and feelings that arise if the new posture proves inadequate as well. This is all part of the fabric of studying yourself.

With the intention of sitting through their pain, people often ask which pain can be safely ignored and which pain is actually damaging to the body. It's difficult to make any hard-and-fast calls in a book, but in general, nerve pain (tingling, numbness, aching down the leg) ought to be accommodated. Whenever my foot "goes to sleep," a variant of nerve compression, I contract my buttock muscles to release the nerve and get blood flowing again down into the foot. This requires such a slight adjustment that an onlooker would probably be unaware of my movement. If your knees or ankles get chronically swollen, sitting cross-legged might be too hard on your joints. Stretching exercises might solve the problem. If your lower back starts to ache or get tired, try breathing into the vertebrae there to relieve and slightly stretch them. If you don't feel nerve pain radiating down your leg, it is probably all right to put up with a tired back as long as it recovers as soon as your meditation period is over. Again, you should be able to find exercises to strengthen your back muscles, which will mean less pressure on the vertebrae.

With the aim of continuing to develop your ability to sit through almost everything, some meditation teachers recommend that you feel the impulse to move three times before you actually obey it and adjust your posture. I agree, because if you adopt such a rule, you'll still get a good idea of your mind's response to pain, but it won't be a protracted and potentially debilitating struggle.

STABILITY AND VULNERABILITY

When we do meditation, formal or informal, we are developing stability and vulnerability at the same time. Our posture and our commitment to being present for everything, no matter what comes up, cultivate our stability. Paying attention to what comes up and relaxing into the thoughts and feelings that arise develop our vulnerability. If we err on the side of stability, never opening ourselves to the unexpected or unwanted, we become rigid, impervious. If we are too vulnerable, carried away with every stray thought and feeling, unable to recognize them as transient, we go crazy. The postures presented in the preceding section—all of them some variant on keeping the lower body stable and the spine as straight as possible—are the perfect practice to find our way in this realm: our thinking minds give way to softness, receptivity, right in the middle of our strength. Our open awareness provides a sense of ease for body and mind that furthers our commitment and strengthens our posture. Effort and ease, stability and openness, are completely integrated. This is the effortless effort spoken of by the ancients.

When we are very stable in our formal meditation, we feel like a mountain on which plants grow, animals forage, humans hike, and storms rage, but none of this disturbs the essential imperturbability of the mountain and its rootedness as an integral part of the earth itself. When we are vulnerable, awash in emotion, we feel more like the surface of a lake, its glassy countenance rent by the constant hubbub of fish splashing, turtles swimming, motorboats roaring, and humans shouting and playing. But even with all this commotion on top, the darkness and quiet of the depths remain undisturbed. The fish move silently; the plants grow soundlessly but surely, extending their tendrils in the hush. This, too, is stability, imperturbability. Thich Nhat Hanh wrote that "When mind has taken hold of mind, dispersed mind is true mind." When we're aware that we are spaced-out, absent-minded, does that mean we are present in the moment or oblivious?

Demon, or hindrance, meditation and shikan taza develop stability in meditation because they cultivate the sense of connection to everything—not only to ease and serenity but to all the thoughts and emotions in our minds, including those we don't want. A feeling of connection contributes enormously to stability. The primal connections—to our breath, the sensations of our body, our thoughts and emotions—give us a ground of being. They make up our primordial "home," the home we find when we leave our ordinary home, our parents' house, the region where we grew up, or even our current residence. They are where we come back to, moment after moment. In this way, our true home is not anywhere in particular but everywhere: every thought we have, every sensation we feel, every breath we take. We are always at home.

A particularly primal connection for humans is to the breath. When I was much younger, I was frequently assailed by terrifying thoughts that made me panicky. I also used to take psychedelic

drugs, which sometimes eased my fears but at other times intensified them so badly that I could become so confused, I didn't
know whether I was alive or not. Eventually I discovered that I
could use my breath as a criterion for survival. No matter how
crazed or frightened I was, how far I had strayed from my ordinary consciousness, I felt for my breath. Sometimes that was all I
had when everything else was unfamiliar. Ever since, whenever I
have had to help other people through some great psyche-shat-
tering upheaval—bad drug trips, terminal medical diagnoses, debilitating grief—that's always where I direct them: toward breath.
When you put your hands on your diaphragm and feel something moving there, that's an incontestable reference point, the
tether for your life at that moment. If you are willing to put up
your flag there, to stake your claim and make your homestead
there, you will develop the stability to face everything else.

After sitting meditation for an entire day, a woman told me
that she had now embarked on another way of life. When I appeared startled, she explained that she had realized a very bad
habit pattern that appeared to be responsible for much of her
stress. In every situation in which another human being was involved, she revved up her mind and body to meet the situation.
Once her performance was over, she would return to her comforting nest of self and go numb until the next demand on her
from the outside. Not only did she speed up for her job, but it
occurred on very subtle levels, every time she was with another
person or even whenever the phone rang. What happened during her day of meditation was that she realized she could make
breath the center of her life rather than her fear of not being
pleasing. As she put it, she could make a "lifetime commitment
to something more primal" than her need to please: her breath.
This touched me very much. A shift of this magnitude can create
tremendous stability in both your meditation practice and your
life.

This is a good reason to develop the habit of doing formal
meditation. Your mind then knows it will have a regular time to
settle and watch the mad world (the *internal* mad world, that is)
go by. The patience you cultivate through periodically focusing

your attention and observing your habits without criticism contributes greatly to the growth of stability in your meditation practice. You need this kind of consistency to be able to sit through summer heat, itches and twitches, emotional turmoil, whatever arises in your mind and body, with steadiness and energy. It's much easier to foster this steadfastness in formal meditation than when you are racing around trying to cope with the demands of a hectic life.

A meditation student confided to me that he felt enervated by his cautionary approach to his life and the ponderous, extended decision-making process that every new step seemed to require: getting a promotion, applying to grad school, finding a new roommate. He told me that for a long time, he had mistaken his general emotional numbness for equanimity, but in long periods of meditation, like a day or two, he began to understand that a whole layer—possibly many layers—of pain and grief awaited him whenever he was quiet and not focused on his usual concerns. It was like tender little shoots of grass growing up through the cracks in the sidewalk. Although he was terrified of whatever emotional chaos might be in there, he found himself wanting to have a real life, a vital life, every bit as much as he wanted to feel that he had some control over things. He was asking me to give him support while he was delving into his pain and chaos. He was quite sophisticated psychologically and knew that he needed a friend beside him to launch such an exploration.

Allowing feelings like these to arise, as he was committing himself to do, takes a great deal of stability: you have to actually feel your bottom on the cushion or the ground; you have to feel that one breath is followed by another; you have to feel connected to some aspects of life and want to be even more connected; you have to have faith that you will continue sitting right here and that whatever comes up will not overwhelm you or drive you crazy. The courage or fearlessness that allows this kind of resolve is developed by stability, the commitment to facing life with a stable base and an erect spine, whatever your posture.

IN GENERAL, it is very important to be patient with yourself when you are beginning a meditation practice. You are attempting something that is inherently very difficult: breaking old habits. And these habits aren't even as blatant as biting your fingernails or smoking cigarettes. They're habits of mind. The rule of thumb is that it takes ten thousand times to notice that you have a bad habit, ten thousand more times to catch yourself doing it, and ten thousand more times to substitute an alternative behavior. The ancients who derived this dictum understood the coercive power of habit. With this practice, you will begin to as well.

11

SWALLOWING THE WHOLE WORLD

◌

COPING WITH STRESS

An article in the *San Francisco Chronicle* points out that increasing numbers of American workers have stress levels that threaten their health and well-being. The American Medical Association estimates that up to 70 percent of all patients seen by general practice doctors come with symptoms directly related to unrelieved stress. Stress is also among the top ten reasons Americans miss work, according to the Occupational Safety and Health Administration. A doctor at an Arizona medical center is quoted as saying that people don't realize what stress does to the body. It's a factor in protracted colds, intestinal problems, anxiety, insomnia, back strains, carpal tunnel syndrome, high blood pressure, fatigue, depressions, migraines, weakened immune systems, ulcers, blood clots, chest pains, and heart attacks.

One of today's biggest concerns is how to deal with stress. We call it by many names: job burnout, information overload, posttraumatic stress, the rat race, what have you. The basic problem is, how do we live our lives, put food on the table, raise our children with the advantages we want them to have, maintain our health, provide for our retirement, and finally—whew!—live lives that are so satisfying that on our deathbeds, we can look back without regret and say, "Well, I had a full, rich life in which I lived every moment!"?

Life has never been easy for any creature, including those of us with human bodies, but we have even more to cope with in our age of anxiety than the usual predators, pain and sickness, and the acquisition of food and shelter. We live in a culture that is profoundly materialistic. Work that produces goods and services and the consumption of those goods and services are the most important things. Given this disproportionate emphasis on tangibles, we have gradually allowed our primal connections to other things, like our bodies and our subtle feelings, to be discounted and mechanized. Interpersonal relationships have been compromised by the cultural need to achieve and compete. Spiritual ties, which I will define as a belief in some reality beyond the material world, have for many people been severed altogether. We don't take very seriously the impulses we may feel toward the satisfaction of personal and spiritual needs; we don't allow time for contemplation or seek solitude for reflection and renewal.

Our embrace of recent technological developments has created a situation in which we can never get disconnected from our work responsibilities. We can be E-mailed, faxed, beeped, phoned, and paged anywhere. Ironically, all this communication has not made us feel more in touch with each other. Messages on our answering machines and numbers on our beepers are often felt as annoyances, just more straws on the pile when we're already stressed out and strung out, rather than as opportunities to relate to another human being, to share our burdens and relieve stress.

For many of us, the result of this isolation from all the emotional and spiritual sustenance that mattered to countless generations of human beings is that when a crisis disrupts our daily lives and forces us back upon our resources, we are shocked and dismayed to find we don't have many! We have no anchor, no ground, to guide us. We frantically search outside ourselves, running to doctors, gurus of all sorts, radio advice programs, and people we know for answers only our own hearts can provide. Since we long ago lost touch with our hearts—our deep yearnings and needs—we can't figure out what is important in these new straits. We can't tell what should have priority and thus what we should do next.

How Meditation Can Help

The most important step in breaking free of a life dominated by stress and anxiety is to be present for what is actually happening rather than to be swept away with our ideas about what may happen to us later. For example, I'm always fairly hysterical before I give a public talk. But when I actually get up at the podium and look out over the audience, I see smiles here and there, I hear the rustle of clothing as people settle into their seats, and I feel something that must be the warm "rays" of people's attention entering my chest. I calm down. Then the dance begins: the vivid exchange of energy between me and my audience. I hear my voice over the mike, and I see the wave of it hit people's bodies. The impact of my words on them is visible. Their upper bodies either close up or take me in. So despite my pre-event terror, it turns out that public speaking energizes and delights me. It's as if the fear I was feeling beforehand creates energy that is then plowed back into my nervous system as a heightened awareness. I actually think of giving public talks as an altered state.

So there is a difference between actually living an event, being open to all the details of its immediacy, and thinking about it beforehand, just imagining it. Our heads know our inadequacies very well. When we're present with our bodies, receiving somatic information (which our intellects may not even be aware of), some kind of magic happens. The situation becomes much fuller and assumes an integrity our heads could not even comprehend. So much stress comes from our imaginings, our abstract ideas about situations, rather than the reality of them. Of course, plenty of stress comes from the reality of them as well, which is why we ought to refine our worries to the point that they consist of emotional reactions to real rather than projected circumstances (such as if the house really did burn down).

Thoughts about my future mobility crop up and worry me

since I have already lost some function to rheumatoid arthritis. I start to wonder, When will I be confined to a wheelchair? When will it be too painful to hold a grandchild on my lap? I swear that these projections onto the future cause me more anguish than the actual pain and disability I experience at any given moment! This is why it is so important to set up your camp in the present moment and to give yourself permission to not know what will happen next or how you will deal with the next moment. At least right now, you are alive and coping with what is here before you.

Ironically, when you give yourself permission to be out of control (in the sense that who knows what you might do if you sink into the present with all your senses and feelings available to you, right?), time slows down so dramatically that you have a heightened sense of being in control. This is because you become aware of the more subtle aspects of the situation—your own physical sensations, perhaps your heart beating, your cheeks flushing, a look on someone's face, the inflection in a voice, the body language of fear or aggression. The great thing is that since you noticed all this, you now have a wide range of options in terms of your reaction. When you pay attention to what is happening right now, all of your resources come into the present with you; they're not suppressed by the habits of thought that usually block them. So the odds of your handling the situation with skill and positively influencing the flow of events are maximized, not minimized, by your conscious presence.

It may be very scary to picture yourself in a stressful moment—say, an argument with a coworker—present and vulnerable with no road map to follow, no automatic straitjacket to keep your emotions in check. But in reality, in the moment when you're actually arguing with that coworker, you realize you don't have to suppress your feelings and thoughts to prevent yourself from going out of control. You can feel threatened and hurt and angry without doing anything that will jeopardize your job. Being conscious in the present, you can see your feelings and thoughts for what they are: feelings and thoughts. They don't necessarily have to lead to action. You are free to think any thoughts, feel any feelings you want; you are not free to haul off and punch your coworker. You are perfectly capable of making this distinction.

If, in these moments of stress, you can manage to refer to your breath for even a second, it will change your reference point in the whole situation. You get a split-second break and thus a chance to return to the stressful situation just perceptibly refreshed, but even that tiny bit of refreshment is enough for you to see your options. Not only that, the short pause for your breath sets up the next pause for your breath and then the next pause after that. In a flicker of your mind's eye, your breath provides the perspective to continue being present when all the forces of habit are pulling you toward an automatic response.

Replacing your automatic reactions to stress with an attitude of open awareness is not easy. It takes a great deal of practice and cultivation. You will have to do it over and over again before your meditation muscle is strong enough to take you through an entire crisis, even if the crisis only lasts a few minutes. At first, you will be lucky to interrupt your torrent of reactivity with a single breath, one moment of open awareness when you suddenly register your heartbeat, an acid taste in your mouth, or any of your physiological responses to crisis. After you have done this breath check-in many times in many different situations, you will develop a great deal of faith in your ability to hold your ground in difficult situations—not necessarily with the wisdom of Solomon, but with your very own intelligence and sanity, to which you will have greater access since you have started looking past your habit patterns for options.

In time, you get to know what to expect from yourself, what words terrify you, what situations render you feeling helpless, what you say when you are angry, what kind of ground you need under you to feel solid, and with that knowledge comes a willingness to bring all of yourself into difficult circumstances. You come to regard yourself as a reasonable person doing your best, and so you deserve the consideration and respect due every being, even from yourself.

Years ago, when I was in the first throes of my bout with rheumatoid arthritis, I walked with a marked limp, which made my pace very slow. Our urban neighborhood was a dangerous one then, populated with drug dealers and gangs. One night, I had no choice but to walk the short distance from the trolley to my apartment with my three-year-old son. Suddenly I heard hard footsteps behind us, and as I was turning around to look, I felt myself grabbed from behind, my head forced back and my neck in a choke hold. "Grab the purse!" my captor shouted at his companion. The other man immediately started pulling on my shoulder bag. I held onto it reflexively without thought.

Then everything really slowed down as I entered some kind of altered state. The first thing I was aware of was my heart beating so hard it filled my ears. I could also feel my own breathing, which was oddly deep and comforting. There was no doubt I was alive, despite this unforeseen setback. Finally I was aware of my captor's body, warm against my back with an arm around my neck. He had my head pulled back so there was nothing in partic-ular to look at; I could see a treetop. I felt the anxious tugging going on at my left side as one of the men struggled to pull my purse away from me. "Let go of the purse!" the one holding me shouted into my ear. Even though I was holding on to my purse with all my might, having crossed my arms together around the strap, I wondered why their indisputably superior strength wasn't allowing them to prevail against a crippled woman. If the man holding me had tightened his arm around my neck even slightly, I would have choked and relinquished my purse just as reflexively as I had begun holding on to it. But he didn't seem to realize this advantage; his hold on me was oddly distracted. I understood from this that I was actually the more focused one and that I might be able to keep my purse, as their efforts became increas-ingly frenetic and ineffective.

Suddenly, as I was actually beginning to relax, I heard my son cry out. "Oh, my God," I thought, "they're turning their attention on him!" I immediately let go of my purse. My captor grabbed the purse, dropped me like a stone, and the two of them took off running fast. No longer at all concerned with our mug-gers, I looked at my son. He was fine, just upset. I realized how little real time must have elapsed. Ethan probably started crying as soon as he apprehended the danger. Because he was a country commune child with no TV or familiarity with violence, it must have taken him several seconds to understand that other people might actually hurt us. I couldn't get up off the ground by myself, but people began pouring out of neighboring houses. By this, I understood that some of the sounds accompanying the mugging must have been audible to others as well. I was impressed by how heightened my awareness of my own body and the body pressed against me from behind had been.

Typically, mugging victims collapse or tremble afterward as they experience the fear they felt in the situation. I had no such feelings. I wondered whether it was because after the first second or so, I was in such contact with my mugger's body that the fear disappeared. I knew him so intimately. I knew I would not be hurt. It wasn't until I feared for Ethan, whom I couldn't actually see, that I reappraised the situation. I have never forgotten the feelings I had during that evening because I was so impressed that the intense immediacy of the situation yielded up a tremendous amount of accurate information. Every nuance of the man's body, and the unwavering stability of my own, was processed by my senses. Of course, in an unusual situation like this, we don't have to practice mindfulness of our breath and body sensations. It comes to us unbidden. When our adversary is our boss, our mate, or a friend, we have to direct our attention to our breath and body; it probably won't go there by itself. I tell you this story to demonstrate the amount of information available to you in a stressful situation when you tune in to many levels of it.

MINDFULNESS
THE EVERYDAY-LIFE MEDITATION

Most people take up a meditation practice not to become yogic adepts but in order to cultivate the mental agility to deal with pain and stress more easily. They may wish to have their full psychic resources available to them, to feel expansive and energetic, open to all the world has to offer, even when faced with personal crisis and the world's insoluble woes.

Formal meditation practice doesn't actually mean very much unless it generalizes to our everyday lives. Many of us develop skill in sitting still and a remarkable ability to concentrate, but what are these meditation skills worth if they are not put into service to broaden and deepen our world rather than narrow it to a single point? Few of us have the opportunity or inclination to inhabit a monk's cave; most of us must cope with the fast, furious pace of our materialistic culture. A coworker's lack of co-operation, a job layoff, a mate's diagnosis of cancer, a traffic snarl that keeps us from making the plane—this is where the serenity and willingness to be present for everything, good and bad, that is cultivated in formal meditation will be truly tested. Formal and informal meditation practice complement each other. If you commit yourself to doing both, formal practice will give your mind a place to practice stability more consistently; informal practice in your daily life will offer the true test of holding your ground and yet being open to all that comes. When you are work-ing on your computer against a deadline and your small child enters the room, can you turn and give her your full attention before going back to work?

In order to be willing to develop your ability to be present in your everyday life, you might ask yourself why you are not more present now. What conditions put you on "automatic pilot"? What emotions underlie your "numb" states of mind? Do you get excessively preoccupied with compulsive thoughts about what you have to get done because your emotional life is painfully cha-otic or because it's just a habit that you haven't questioned? It's not easy to break the habits of mind that keep you imprisoned in a fog of routine or a cage of vehement conviction. At first, at-tempting to be more aware of your life is like sticking a frail pole into a rushing river. The river of obliviousness swirls around your pole, threatening to carry it away. You have one moment of pres-ence in a day or week of unconsciousness. But with practice, the pole gets fatter and stouter and longer. Especially if you are in great and constant pain or under crushing stress, it behooves you to develop enough awareness to locate the spaces in the pain or stress where you can live with relative ease—the cracks in the concrete where the grass grows up through. If you think of yourself as constantly one way (in pain or depressed or anxious), try paying close attention to how you feel. You may be surprised to see how much your attitude fluctuates on a subtle level over a day's time. The fact that there is some fluctuation implies that you might begin to get a handle on, or gain some control over, your state of mind by noticing what affects it.

There are many different kinds of meditation practice that will help you cultivate the ability to be present in stressful situations. Body awareness meditations are particularly useful because they develop your ability to return to your physical body again and again, whatever the circumstance in which you find yourself, until you intuitively understand that your body is the ground of your consciousness; you are not just a talking head. Awareness of body, breath, or sense impressions is a very grounding and settling reference point for the attention because they are not involved in the gaining and losing judgments of our day-to-day lives.

Stabilizing the self in the body, doing routine tasks from the point of view of the body, can be a tremendously comforting refuge from the continual flow of stress-producing thoughts through the mind. I myself especially enjoy folding laundry with my attention on the laundry itself because of the comforting smell of freshly washed cloth. Even though it's somewhat painful to my arthritic hands, I find washing a big load of dishes the day after a dinner party very reassuring. Not only am I flooded with memories of my companions of the night before and the witty things that were said, but since I married late in life, the majority of my kitchen things are wedding presents and are still intact. I think of each plate and serving dish as layered with pleasant memories of people I still know and some I have not seen for years. And if there has been a break, I feel the melancholy twinges of regret, still very sweet when they blend with the hot, soapy water and the smell of cooking odors from the night before.

Another stable reference point to anchor you when you are overwhelmed is your sense data, the constant stream of information you are always receiving from your eyes, ears, nose, taste buds, and skin sensors but of which you are usually unaware because it is so mundane. To focus on sense impressions without concepts or judgment is to enter a world so rich, so varied, so inherently fascinating that you might wonder how you chose to spend most of your time in the world of thoughts and concepts. When I give workshops for people in great pain, I turn them loose in a garden with instructions to meditate on the impressions from each of their senses in turn. I do this specifically to demonstrate how close at hand is delight they might have overlooked in their preoccupation with their pain. It is very helpful to practice with the anchors of breath, body sensation, and sense impression in your everyday life. The mind learns that there is a place it can go that opens up a reality beyond thought and opinion, worry and judgment. If you introduce this kind of consciousness into your daily life on a regular basis, you increase your odds of being able to return there when things get out of whack.

The following mindfulness practices are designed specifically for infusing your everyday life activities with spaciousness, awareness, and ease. If you take the trouble to do them with patience and determination, you will fatten your awareness pole in the midst of the rushing stream of your typical thoughts, worries, fantasies, compulsions, and personal opinions. Since it is not easy to hold up this pole in the face of years of habit and virtually no support in the general culture, you would be helped tremendously if, at the same time that you develop some ability to pay attention to your activity, you also cultivate patience and kindness toward yourself and admiration for your efforts.

- Eat one meal, or part of a meal, with mindful attention every day. This means, give great attention to the movements involved as you eat: cutting, lifting the fork, chewing, your pattern of chewing, swallowing, and so forth. Give full attention to the taste of the food as it enters your mouth, after it has been in your mouth for a time, is chewed, and swallowed.

Notice your thoughts, sensations, and emotions about the food and your activity.

- Every day at (fill in your own time) and (fill in another time later in the day), notice what posture your body is in—whether it's lying, sitting, standing, walking—and whether it is comfortable.
- Select three everyday tasks a week—washing dishes, dusting, and folding clothes, for instance—and do them mindfully.
- Notice how you treat your spouse and children. Are you less polite and considerate to them than to anyone else? If you are, examine what habits or beliefs allow you to behave less graciously to the ones you most love than to a relative stranger.
- Keep a diary or make a list of everything that comforts you when you are miserable—which objects (sweets, drugs, charms) and which experiences (music, company, trash reading, TV)—and notice what is happening just before you reach for them.
- Use your bathing as a meditation: be attentive to every movement; place your attention on every part of your body; be mindful of each stream of water on your body.
- Devote one day of the week entirely to mindfulness of everything you do. Begin while lying in bed and wear something (a ring, a bracelet, an article of clothing) to remind you of your intention during the day.
- When you wake up, use the seconds before you get out of bed to gently inhale and exhale three breaths, following the breaths closely and feeling your bodily sensations.
- Track one pleasant and one unpleasant experience every day, noting (1) when you were aware of the nature of each experience (during it? afterward?); (2) how your body felt during it; (3) what mood, thoughts, or additional feelings you had; (4) what thoughts or feelings you now have about it.
- Be aware of feelings you don't want for a day, a week, a month, without trying to change them, get away from them, or even express them. Stay with them and try to hold them

in "meditative equipoise." If you can't stay with them, notice where you go.

- When you first open your eyes in the morning, observe how you put your personality together for the day: thought by thought, identity by identity, role by role, until your idea of yourself is in place.
- While vacuuming, move from your body's point of view. Feel your lower body joints and muscles support the upper body as you manipulate the vacuum cleaner. Focus on distributing your lower body weight over your feet, knees, hips, and lower back. When you bend to get under furniture, breathe as you curl your spine forward and let your neck hang loosely in front of your chest.
- When you ride your bike, try making sure that your legs alone are doing the work and that your hips and back are completely relaxed. Your pedal stroke should come from your thigh and lower leg muscles rather than your lower back. Make the ease of your body, rather than the destination of your ride, your priority.
- While you are walking—either a short distance (to the photocopier or the refrigerator) or a long way (to work or in the park for recreation and exercise)—try the following:

Count the number of steps you take per breath, considering a whole breath—inhalation, exhalation, and pause in between—as a unit. Focus on the sensations in your body as you shift your weight from one foot to the other. There will be a tremendous amount of feeling from the bottom of your feet, along your legs, up to your hips and lower back. Think "Muscle and bone, muscle and bone," becoming aware of what takes place in your body as you walk.

Become aware of one sense impression in particular or of all those that come in through your eyes, ears, nose, mouth, and skin. What do you see? Smell? Hear? Taste? Feel on your skin? Try to experience these sensations in a raw way, not labeling what the stimulation is (a car passing, a flower, what you had for lunch).

As an adjunct to the preceding mindfulness practice, notice whether these sensations are pleasant or unpleasant.

Pay attention to all the sounds you hear, whether internal or external. Resist labeling their source; it doesn't matter. Just experience their arising and passing, their overlap, their individuality.

Try seeing everything that comes in through your eyes as simple color and form, not in terms of concepts like what the object is, how it's used, and so on. Notice how really difficult it is to see objects apart from their function.

- Whenever you encounter another person during the day, try the following:

  Tune in to your breath at least once and notice whether your breathing is deep or shallow, fast or slow, or whether you are holding your breath.

  If that person is telling you his troubles, tune in to your own feelings and your body reactions several times during the interaction.

  While the person is telling you his troubles, practice resisting the impulse to "advise" him, offering him your full attention instead.

  While you are telling your troubles to someone else, tune in to your own breath and body feelings several times during the telling.

  When you tell your troubles, practice being clear about what kind of reaction you wish for from your friend. Notice whether you scan her face to find it or modify your behavior to get it.

These suggestions are my favorites, but there are many more in these helpful books: *Full Catastrophe Living,* by Jon Kabat-Zinn; *A Path with Heart,* by Jack Kornfield; and *The Miracle of Mindfulness,* by Thich Nhat Hanh. My own book *Arthritis: Stop Suffering, Start Moving: Everyday Exercises for Body and Mind* contains a plethora of mindfulness exercises in which the sensations of the body serve as a reference point while doing daily tasks: dressing, housework, and recreation.

As you gradually develop the skill to deliberately pay attention, the awareness that you might choose to cultivate in your everyday life relates to whatever you personally regard as your primary suffering. If you suffer chronic pain, it might be most advantageous to focus on the movements you make in your routine activities that cause you to feel better or worse. Does it make your hip hurt less if you swing your leg out when you walk? What kinds of movements affect your pain? If you are depressed, it might be most useful to focus on your energy level. What raises or lowers it? Certain thoughts, interactions with certain people? If you start to get wound up tighter and tighter from pressure and stress, it might help to locate the specific thought that kicks off your spiral of fear. As mentioned earlier, if you think of yourself as constantly one way (in pain or depressed or stressed-out), you might be surprised to see how much you fluctuate on a subtle level over a day's time, and you might consider how you could begin to manipulate that fluctuation by noticing what affects it. It is enormously helpful for you to discover what it is you call suffering, what needs are being frustrated when you are suffering, and how you might satisfy those needs.

A nurse in one of my stress-reduction classes asked for advice about what I consider a pivotal dilemma for many people: "My job is so terrible that if I were actually present during it, as you recommend, I would go insane. It's only the numbness that makes my situation bearable at all. Why should I cultivate mindfulness in such a situation?"

This often happens in the helping professions: nursing, family therapy, drug counseling, social work with abused or homeless children. Of course, the situations such workers deal with are horrible, unspeakable, unbearable. What role does awareness have under such circumstances? Doesn't it only increase your suffering? Yes, of course, it does. And this is why developing the stability that can be cultivated through formal meditation practice is very important to people in these professions. You need to be very grounded to allow the extreme suffering of innocent people to enter you, perceive it, feel it, and then let it pass out of you. If you block the suffering in front of you and become numb in order to protect yourself, you're not much use to those who turn to you for help. It's very important to all of us that our suffering register with someone, that someone take it seriously. It's most helpful to feel suffering and let it pass through you, not sticking anywhere.

I think what meditation and mindfulness do for people in these situations is widen their weave—that is, awareness without judgment makes the openings in their bodies large enough for enormous amounts of suffering to be registered and then pass through, leaving no trace. The suffering is burned up completely in the moment it's felt. When I feel this in my own body, it's as if my weave were so wide, there's so much space between the fibers of my tissue, my insides must resemble the loosely interlaced potholders kindergartners make at school and proudly present to their parents.

You can't discharge the suffering, allow it to pass through, unless you're paying attention, vibrating, pulsating with the waves of suffering you feel, aware of your own breathing and grounded by it and the sense impressions impinging on you. Being settled in your breath and body makes it easier to settle also in your mind, which reels with its projections into the future and its fears of the present.

My husband has one of these burnout jobs, the kind that people break down at after about three years, and they move on, some with post-traumatic stress syndrome. He's a "street therapist" and has been working with homeless people for more than ten years. He tells me that faced with the incomprehensible suffering he sees every day on the part of sick people, old people, disabled people, crazy people, women, and children, it's most important for him to deal just with what is happening right in front of him, with no thought of what will happen, even ten minutes from now.

He might spend three hours finding a bed for a homeless person for that night because she is sick and exhausted from being on the street. If he invests himself in whether she actually gets herself to that bed some four hours later, he is doomed to worry and frustration. If he finds one of his clients dead on the sidewalk from a beating or an overdose after having put weeks of therapy and social services together to help him, he can only grieve for the person he cared about. He can't emotionally afford to harbor feelings of hopelessness about the effectiveness of his efforts. He must experience those feelings and let them pass. While he was administering the therapy and setting up the social services for that client, he couldn't afford to ponder what might happen—or even was likely to happen—to thwart his efforts to get the client off the streets. Everything he does must be for its own sake, for the exchange made in that very moment he and his client meet. He once described the emotional tone of his job to me as "trying to pull people from a shipwreck with the Nazis firing on you." Here are some excerpts from his journal:

Woke up this AM with the unwanted thought that Anita has killed herself or managed to get herself murdered. I feel light-bodied and irritated. I sit and stare at the walls, take an hour to get up the nerve to go to Anita's hotel. I finally get up and go to the Tenderloin. Anita answers her door all cheerful. So much for my fabled intuition. More like burnout, I guess. Anita will forever be a problem for someone. She's pushing forty and is a third-generation prostitute. She grew up in Houston. When she was three years old, her mother set her on fire. Child Protective Services later returned her to her mom. . . .

Thomas comes into the clinic with his own peculiar brand of unpleasantness. The implanted radios are going full-blast, sending him constant messages about the conspiracies against him. I find out that he did seven years in the pen for fucking his seven-year-old daughter, the number being a sort of coincidental quid pro quo. I think they should have locked up the poor, crazy motherfucker for life. "She really wanted it," he tells me, "I know she did." I find out later that he once hit another child so hard upside the head that he killed her and did little or no time for it. Today he is making sure I know that he is closely associated with Jesse James. I tend to believe it. I cannot help but imagine the hell he lives in and, even worse, the suffering he has put on others. It does not surprise me, however, that he is running around loose. Your parking meter runs out of time—count on swift reprisal by the government in the form of at least a ticket. Rape and kill a child, do some time, plead crazy, which you certainly are, and you're eligible for free legal assistance, disability benefits, and state-subsidized health care. Am I bitter and confused? Am I moving to the right? The idea of just not thinking things through is at times very, very attractive. . . .

I walk down Sixth Street from Market to Howard with Marian. It is bright, smoggy; the street is noisy with traffic. The sidewalks are crammed with crackheads, speed freaks, drunks, crazies, and cripples. The energy is intense, and there is a sharp, freewheeling hostility swirling around in the air; no one is in a good mood. The piss smell in the alleys and doorways is so thick that I keep thinking that I see the fumes. . . . Maybe things are just generally turning meaner. There are lots of racial overtones. Everybody has their mind made up. There is less and less room for maneuvering. I find myself angry at all the meanness in the world. And sometimes I am just plain exasperated, and I do not feel like being fucked with.

What I admire about my husband's attitude toward his experiences is that he has strong emotional reactions but no judgments about those reactions. He may have opinions about how things should be and how human beings should treat each other, but he does not do his work from these opinions. He sees what is in front of him, and he commits himself to it without holding back.

Although my husband's recollections may be an extreme example of the need to let strong feelings arise and disappear without attachment to them, with dangerous psychological consequences from holding onto them, we can apply his insights to the stress and pain of our own lives because with an attitude of impression without judgment, we are all capable of reaching beyond our ideas of suffering and delight into the realm of living fully each moment as it comes. As Zen teacher Kanshi Sosan wrote in his long poem "Shinshinming," "The Great Way is not difficult for those who have no preferences. When love and hate are both absent everything becomes clear and undisguised. Make the smallest distinction, however, and heaven and earth are set infinitely apart." Should my husband indulge in the smallest expectation or the glimmer of a hope, heaven and earth would be set infinitely apart.

Mindfulness meditation in our everyday lives is not the practice of self-improvement; it is forgetting the self in our absorption in our immediate activity. Forgetting the self is just doing a task with no self-consciousness sticking to the action. The voice of "I am doing this," "I am doing that" is drowned out by the awareness of the body sensations involved in the task; the swinging door of breath-in, breath-out; the thoughts necessary to organize and project the next steps in the task; the sense impressions of our immediate environment. When we can do our work and relate to other people without constantly constructing and maintaining a rigid identity, the perception of our daily lives as spacious and full of possibilities expands to include our mundane suffering.

OBSTACLES TO EVERYDAY AWARENESS
OPINION, PRECONCEPTION, AUTOMATIC PILOT

Why isn't it easier to practice the art of being in the present? It should be the most natural thing in the world to just be in the moment, as animals are. Why is it so difficult for us to keep our full attention on what we're doing and feeling right now? Why do we prefer our fantasies and projections? Why do we need days and weeks and months of practice counting our breaths in order to feel alive? Isn't it our birthright?

The answer lies partly in our cultural emphasis on thoughts to the exclusion of feelings and sensations. Because we have been educated to attach so much importance to our ability to formulate thoughts and concepts, we tend to live our lives dominated by personal opinion rather than immediate experience. Opinion locks us into ideas about other people based on what they seem to be doing or saying or how they look. Fixed ideas limit what we can do or say, how we can enjoy ourselves or choose mates.

Sometimes preconceived notions so hinder our ability to sense and feel that when we look at something, we see our idea of it rather than the thing itself. For instance, we often think social status when we see a luxury car, or have sexual feelings when we see a heart-shaped box. Preconceptions are how we separate ourselves from actual experience. When we live like this, believing the opinions and preconceptions that set us apart from everything we encounter rather than experiencing our interconnectedness with every other being and thing, we feel pretty isolated. As Joko Beck says in *Everyday Zen,* "All of practice [mindfulness, meditation] is to return ourselves to pure experiencing."

Relying on our preconceptions also encourages us to live our lives on automatic pilot. We get through our days just doing what we did the last time we were in a similar situation. If we don't feel much, we can cope by trotting out our habitual opinion about something every time it presents itself. That way, we can sleep through our lives without nudging ourselves into consciousness. It's so much easier to go into habit mode when we hear a relative's voice on the phone. Since we think of this person as annoying and verbose, we can tune out the conversation. If we hate our jobs, it's so much easier to go on automatic pilot when we reach the workplace. We get through the day, but unfortunately we may have forgotten how to wake up when we get home. It is disquieting, however, to consider the fact that each time something presents itself to us, it is a little different from the time before. If we are on automatic pilot and fail to glimpse the nuances of a situation, we might wake up to find ourselves having lost something precious to us and having no clue why. We didn't realize it was going to be the last time our spouse threatened to leave, our sullen child committed a crime, our high blood pressure led to a stroke.

Automatic Pilot

During the day, notice those moments when you are not paying attention to your activity, when you are on "automatic pilot." What events or circumstances drive you there?

Through meditation and mindfulness, we can develop the ability to go to other parts of ourselves besides our heads; we can cut through the bias toward conceptual thought instilled in us since early childhood. And by cultivating the other facets of our being, we become increasingly able to go around and through the habitual preconceptions and sleepiness that imprison us in narrow corridors. Thus, we enrich and expand our lives exponentially. Although, in God's eyes, both flowers and weeds are living plants with equal value, we love the flowers in our gardens and bestow upon them great care while removing the ignominious weeds. Our attachment to beauty is part of our human nature and therefore worthy of study. But as Shunryu Suzuki points out in his primer *Zen Mind, Beginner's Mind*, "For Zen students a weed is a treasure. With this attitude, life becomes an art."

Sacred and Mundane

1. Think about the objects in your house that you consider "sacred," very precious, that you treat carefully.
2. Then notice how you think about and treat the objects that you consider mundane and take for granted.
3. Practice developing a conscious relationship with one of the objects you take for granted, such as your toothbrush, shoes, fork and spoon, chair. Cultivate an attitude toward one of those objects that more resembles your attitude toward one of your sacred objects.

SWALLOWING THE WHOLE WORLD

In *33 Fingers: A Collection of Modern American Koans*, Case 19, Michael Wenger quotes Woody Allen: "More than any other time in history, mankind faces a crossroads. One path leads to despair and utter hopelessness. The other to total extinction. Let us pray we have the wisdom to choose correctly." Michael Wenger remarks, "Caring leads to frustration. Frustration leads to not caring. Not caring is a mask for not trying, which leads somewhere else. Find out where you are and swallow the whole world."

Swallowing the whole world means living a life centered in your entire perceiving being, beyond your ideas about suffering and delight. Although you may still have those ideas, you are no longer preoccupied with whether it's a bad day or a good one, whether you're gaining or losing, whether your body hurts or you feel great. You just live your life doing everything that you do completely, with your whole heart, for its own sake, not getting into the disliking, the liking, the pleasure or pain, the merit or inadequacy of your performance. Your seat, your stability, is in your activity, whatever you are doing now. The great Zen master Dogen once said, "Realization, neither general nor particular, is effort without desire." He meant that when we understand that we are happiest giving everything our full attention without concern for the outcome, we have had a great insight into the nature of the human heart. I think this also points up the importance of creativity in our lives. "Effort without desire" refers to the attitude of an artist or sculptor creating a work, a poet carefully picking the words that express her feeling, a scientist recording his data, a mother making cookies.

Although our most deeply satisfying activities are those that express our creative impulses, we can also bring this attitude to the activities that we find less than engrossing and imbue them with the same importance that makes our poems and paintings so precious. We can commit our whole selves to them for the time that we spend doing them. We can do the dishes, living through each plate and cup that we scrub with soapy water and make clean; we can fix the faucet with total attention to the wrench and pipe; we can drive home with full awareness of our tired bodies, the other cars around us, the vibes on the highway (did you ever notice how drivers on the same street or highway are mostly all in the same mood?), the music on the CD player; we can have a conversation with a stranger asking directions on the street with the same attention and consideration we would bring to an exchange with a close friend.

With this attitude, any work is meaningful. You are your activity itself, cultivating the doing of work for its own sake, totally immersed in the feelings and sensations of physical movement, creative thought, supporting the flow of life. I always thought that if I'm ever completely crippled by arthritis, unable to do the work I do now, I would like to be a toll collector on one of the many beautiful bridges in the San Francisco Bay area, literally supporting the flow of life. This first occurred to me as a result of an encounter with a toll collector who obviously saw his job this way. Many ancient Zen teaching stories center around toll collectors because of the metaphor of reaching "the other side." I have a modern one to tell.

I had crossed the huge expanse of the Bay Bridge from San Francisco to Oakland to attend a wedding in Emeryville, one of the first exits after you cross the bridge. The Bay Bridge is enormous, consisting of about sixteen lanes, eight eastbound and eight westbound; they are divided by a median strip of office buildings and parked vehicles. I have a terrible sense of direction and am easily flustered by getting disoriented while trying to find my way to a new place. The flow of traffic is not my most creative arena.

I must have missed the Emeryville exit because several exits later, I was lost. Nearly in tears, I exited and turned back toward San Francisco, renewing my search. I scanned every exit sign for hints of Emeryville, but no luck. I found myself starting to go back over the toll bridge to San Francisco. I couldn't stand it. After fortysome years of trying to find my way around and failing every damn time, this particular day, when the stakes were high, my frustration erupted into tearful despair. When I pulled alongside the tollbooth and the collector held out his hand for my dollar, I shook my head. I was hysterical, already late, and giving up hope of seeing my friends married.

"I don't *want* to go back to San Francisco!" I cried. I didn't expect there to be any alternative; I was merely venting, indulging my frustration. To my surprise, the toll collector grinned. "Don't worry about a thing," he said brightly. He got on a microphone and stopped all traffic in both directions on that mighty bridge. The roar of car after car revving its motor after paying the toll stopped completely; it suddenly sounded like a summer day. Pointing to the median strip, the toll collector asked, "Do you see that little driveway there?" It was several lanes away, but I could make out a small break in the grass. "Go through there to get to the other side of the bridge." He finished with a gallant sweep of his arm across the span of lanes toward the median strip.

Though amazed, I managed to thank him extravagantly. Slowly I pulled away from the tollbooth, crossing lane after lane as lines of idling cars waited to be let out of their stalls. I pulled into the little driveway and crossed over to the east side of the bridge, going back toward Oakland. I immediately caught sight of the Emeryville exit and went to the wedding. I told people there what had happened, but nobody believed me. That toll collector was a teacher of the heart for me. How easy it would be to mindlessly take toll after toll until your day is finally over and you can wake up and go home to your real life. His being awake enough to take my suffering seriously had a tremendous impact on me.

I think the quintessential example of doing each thing for its own sake and not for later reward is raising a child. With no realistic hope of gratitude, with no return year after year, without getting the kind of child you want, with no prospect of realizing your dreams through this little person, you change diapers and pay the bills and lend a shoulder to cry on and provide endless psychological support because this is what needs to be done. If your mind ever so much as gathers a twig or two to build a nest of repayment, of gratitude, of being owed something, the misery you are setting up for yourself and your child is crushing, even right there in the moment you think it. If you perform each task involved in care and instruction and affection and protection on your child's behalf, for itself alone because it needs to be done, the experience of raising a child feels very different from trying to raise a little clone of yourself: projecting onto her your unconscious ideals, identifying with her achievements, and using her to increase your self-esteem.

It's probably impossible to raise a child without some of these

entanglements, but I think awareness of our tendencies to identify our personal ideals with our children helps to soften things
up, to make things easier for ourselves and our children. Even
insects and animals do this. They nurture their offspring, exhausting themselves with painful labors, yet in the end have no
reward when their offspring are grown. Our human reward can
be in the doing itself, impelled by our hormones and the satisfaction of connection with our ancient charge.

Strictly speaking, you can't really be committed to anything or
anyone unless you're committed wholeheartedly to everything, à
la "Yes! Yes! And again yes!" Otherwise, you might get mired
forever in the hesitation over whether this is the right moment
to which to commit yourself. You might ask, "How can I commit
myself to someone I don't know or to someone I actually dislike?
How can I commit myself without knowing what's going to happen in the future?" You can't predict the future, you don't like
everybody you meet, but it's not about predicting and liking. It's
about your own life, your own ability to engage yourself, and your
own determination to exploit the possibilities in life to the fullest.
What if you were willing to be disappointed? Even exploited?
Would that make it easier to commit yourself to each moment
and each person? What if you didn't think you had to do anything more about disliking a person than just observing your
thoughts and feelings around the dislike with absolute honesty?

What kind of a commitment is this? Is it something like blindly
leaping into relationships and situations without caution or judgment? In a general sense, yes. If someone on the street has just
engaged you in a conversation, feeling cautious about inviting
him up to your apartment for a drink might be justified. It
doesn't mean you can't engage fully in the conversation you're
having with him now. You only need to draw the boundaries
when it's time to part, with as much presence and conviction as
you had while sharing his life for a conversation. Being judicious
about investing all your savings in a friend's project doesn't mean
you can't give her your full attention as she pitches it to you. You
may wish her all the best with a warm heart but still decide to
turn her down. These are all separate moments, each with its

own concomitant activity. You need not leap into every void; you only need to cultivate some part of you that is willing to do so. This part of you needs to grow to be strong enough to counter the mind that automatically snaps shut with fear.

It's easy to say you're a committed person, but commitment is a hard thing to actually manifest in specific situations. You might believe that your commitment should embrace each person and thing, but in practice, it's hard enough to greet your mate with openness and goodwill at the end of a tough workday. The first step (and the next several thousand after that) is to vow to take good care of everything in your way and then notice what your obstacles are: what thoughts and feelings and judgments interfere with your wholehearted commitment to be present for everything and everyone. Basically, commitment is doing each thing you do, moment after moment; inspecting all your resistance, moment after moment; observing your tendency to zonk out in certain situations, moment after moment. All that resistance and judgment ("She's not worthy of my wholehearted commitment") are part of your commitment to everything there is.

Without Reluctance

Try going through a whole day doing each thing without reluctance. When feelings of resentment or reluctance come up around an activity or a task or a communication, embrace those, too, as part of your openness, your commitment to everything.

Commitment grows as a muscle does, by being exercised. Again, I quote Zen master Kanshi Sosan from his poem "Shinshinming": "Do not search for the truth; only cease to cherish opinions. . . . Obey your own nature and you will walk freely and undisturbed."

When we are able to sink beneath our ideas and opinions into the immediacy of our actual experience, we are no longer preoccupied with gaining and losing. When we are aware of our bodily sensations and raw sense impressions, there is nothing further to look for, no directions, no reason, no expectations. At the moment when our conceptual organizing principles give way to our tactility, we have to be exactly here. Doing each thing for its own sake. Being present right now, right here, giving our activity our whole heart and being, focusing on this endeavor, whatever we are doing, whether it's cooking a meal, handling a project at work, or having an encounter with another person. Doing each thing for its own sake, being exactly here. Giving our activity our whole heart and being is our greatest challenge and the deepest satisfaction in our lives.

12

ALLOWING YOUR LIFE TO UNFOLD

❧

Pulling out the weeds we give nourishment to the plant. We pull out the weeds and bury them near the plant to give it nourishment. . . . So you should not be bothered by your mind. You should rather be grateful for the weeds, because eventually they will enrich your practice. . . . You will feel how they change into self-nourishment.

—SHUNRYU SUZUKI-ROSHI

OUR FAULTS
THE WEEDS OF ENLIGHTENMENT

IN my healing work with severely arthritic people, I met a woman who had actually been seriously injured by her physical therapist in the hospital where she was recovering from a heart attack. She told me the therapist had constantly driven her to exercise more and more, insisting, "You're not working hard enough. You're not doing enough," until my client damaged her own joints by trying to comply with the therapist's demands. The therapist apparently hadn't noticed that my client was working against her own muscles—that is, the muscle tension due to her resistance set up a physical conflict in her body so that the more she pushed her body to move, the more her contracted muscles were forced to move through their own tension. Such a situation is fertile ground for muscle strain and tissue tears. In my client's case, her muscles were so weak and her connective tissue so tight

that the joints were continually jammed together until the carti-
lage was damaged. She told me she blamed herself because her
instincts initially told her that she shouldn't listen to the therapist
because the therapist was so self-critical. The therapist drove herself relentlessly and therefore had no conception of how hard to
push others. She had no internal standards, only habit—the
habit of constantly pushing—and so her judgment was gravely
impaired.

Now if that therapist had been self-aware enough to realize
that she tended to be a driven, critical person, her whole approach would have been different. Whenever she felt herself driving a patient, she would say to herself, "There's my habit pattern
again. I'll be careful here and notice whether my patient seems
tired or in pain." The therapist would have been taking her habitual tendency toward compulsive behavior into account as a
factor in treating her patients. Plus she would have been treating
herself with understanding and compassion. Her patient would
have benefited on two fronts: the therapist would have modeled
compassion, kindness toward the body, which her patient, in her
compromised physical condition, needed to learn; and the patient could have learned from her therapist a good attitude with
which to do exercises. The therapist, through acknowledging her
own dark side, would have protected someone else from it rather
than precipitate the disastrous consequences brought on by her
ignorance.

Our so-called faults are actually our best opportunities to study
ourselves because we tend to pay attention to aspects of ourselves
that make us unhappy. We can practice observing them and com-
pensating for them to protect others. We can even learn to appreciate and value them. For instance, a tendency to become
angry is very useful in motivating us to put effort into correcting
social injustice. Passivity might become the patience we need to
continue many years of meditation practice. A "fault" can be a
virtue in the right situation.

Because we don't usually like to think of ourselves as selfish or
withholding help from a friend in need, we tend to overrule any
hesitation we feel about being of service. But our resistance to

doing a favor for someone might be worth looking into because it could be our instincts telling us this is the wrong thing to do. I discovered this when a friend asked me to accompany her on a long-distance trip to see a critically ill friend of hers. Her friend was a psychic healer who had healed many people with her strong will and concentration. My friend believed that her friend the healer was dying because she refused to seek medical help, feeling that to do so would discredit her own work. My friend intended to confront her with the harm her ego-based delusion was causing and talk her into going to the hospital. She wanted my support and physical presence.

When she asked me to go with her, I was very ambivalent, to say the least. At first, I thought it was just the personal inconvenience—interrupting my work to take a long trip—and I scolded myself for not being more willing to help a friend, especially in what seemed to be a life-or-death situation for her friend. When I experience a conflict like this, I usually live with the dilemma for a few days until it resolves itself internally. I was guessing that I would decide to go. But instead of my willingness to help getting the upper hand, my resistance to going continued to strengthen until I couldn't even have forced myself to do what my friend had requested. During those few days I was thinking about it, I started looking at the situation with my own eyes, not just accepting my friend's point of view. I realized that I actually thought it was wrong to confront this critically ill woman and force her to acknowledge that her faith in her own healing powers was misplaced and that she was causing her own death by her foolishness. This struck me as unlikely to further her healing. I called my friend and suggested that we think of another tack, that forcing the woman to lose face was not going to be an effective intervention.

The next day, my friend called me to say I had been able to articulate her own misgivings; she now agreed that no one should go to her friend's bed and confront her. She ended up talking to the woman's husband about appealing to her to seek medical help based on his own concern (and he was indeed concerned). This strategy proved effective: the healer responded to her husband's heartfelt request. Our lives are very complex; in order to respond effectively to the situations facing us, it seems to me that we need to respect every feeling we have about those situations.

APPRECIATION FOR OUR OWN MULTIFACETED SELVES

Why is it so hard for many of us to be as generous and kind toward ourselves as we are toward others? Part of the problem may be that if we have high ideals, we feel it is inappropriate to value ourselves as much as we value the feelings of others. This notion is actually based on a misconception about how generosity and kindness toward other people work. It is only when we ourselves feel nourished and bountiful that we are willing to share our bounty freely with others.

Our egos work in a "One for me, one for you" kind of way, keeping track of the distribution of benefits. Because of the way our sense of self works, we need to be very conscious of the limits to our generosity in any particular circumstance, so that the balance between taking care of ourselves and being generous with others does not get seriously out of kilter. If we are too selfish and never go out of our way for anyone else, we get too insular; our energy level goes down. But when we exhaust ourselves on someone else's behalf, that's when we might seek to even the balance on a subconscious level, and we can unintentionally do some pretty severe damage to other people. We are likely to hurt someone else out of unconscious resentment if we think we have made a great deal of unappreciated effort on his or her behalf. If we are emotionally exhausted, we tend to keep people and demands at bay with barely conscious, petty strategies like pretending not to see them or being short with them on the phone or doing what they ask in a perfunctory or even hostile way.

When I feel reluctant to be generous, I often experience it as pressure, anxiety, the stress of not being taken care of. When it gets so bad that I begin to envy my body work clients lying on my massage table being moved and eased by my own fingers, I know that things are seriously out of whack, that my own time to be nourished is past due. Since the massage treatments I get are an inviolable part of my regular schedule and necessary for me to be of any use to anybody else, I suddenly realize that the situation needs my attention. I am giving more care than I am getting. It may be that I'm feeling a little more "arthritic" this week, experiencing some extra emotional stress, having some new transition—anything that tips the scales.

At the point at which you feel you are giving too much and not being restored and refreshed, you begin to be a little less trustworthy in your dealings with others. You may find yourself a little weaker in your resolve to give a project all you can or less likely to give someone else the benefit of the doubt or to be spontaneously kind if there are no rewards for you. It is very important to familiarize yourself with where your limits are so that you can rescue yourself before things advance too far and it takes several weeks or months to bring you back into balance. If your balance is seriously askew, even a tropical vacation will not be enough. You will come back resentful instead of refreshed, surly with a new appreciation of what you could be doing instead of what you have to do.

It might at first be very painful to observe the limits of our own generosity because we wish to think of ourselves as infinitely kind. If we take a good, hard look at ourselves, we might flinch at what we see. It's no fun to recognize the petty corners of ourselves: that we can remember ten years later that so-and-so still owes us five dollars; that we keep score of the favors done for us by our friends and the hurts dealt us by our enemies; that we might reflexively and maliciously hurt someone's feelings if we think he or she has hurt us first. In order to know ourselves well, we must be more committed to increasing our self-knowledge than we are to enjoying our perception of ourselves as noble and pure.

When you have been observing yourself through your meditation and mindfulness practice for a while, you come to understand how multifaceted you are, what a bundle of contradictions and conflicting ideas. If you become very familiar with your own contradictions, you can actually feel very wide and expansive, big enough to contain the most outrageous of paradoxes. Sometimes you might even enlarge someone else's scope by demonstrating how you yourself hold seemingly conflicting ideas. A friend of mine told her gynecologist how much benefit she was deriving from the estrogen he had prescribed for her after menopause, commenting that her hair was shiny again, her skin smooth, her energy level higher. He nodded, pleased, and said, "You have the proper attitude toward hormone replacement therapy." Since she hadn't been aware of any big controversy, she was startled and asked him, "What's another attitude toward hormone replacement?" He said, "Well, a lot of women think you should just age naturally and accept the symptoms of growing older without trying to do anything about them." My friend laughed and said, "Oh, I believe that, too!" When he looked puzzled, she added, "Oh, it's OK—I'm very comfortable with paradox." The exam continued in silence. A few minutes later, he said to her completely seriously, "You know, I admire you very much."

If we try to smooth out these contradictions, to make more sense of ourselves, to be more consistent, we do all these aspects of ourselves a grave injustice by lopping off their elaborate curlicues and baroque ornamentation. Why should all these parts of us be under the domain of our reason, our ability to think logically? Our logical minds are only one part of us, and although they may be the cleverest, they are certainly not the most perceptive, the wisest, or the sanest. We're very complicated beings, and we do our diverse selves a disservice by trying to make them all consistent. Not only do humorlessness and arrogance and acceptance and compassion all exist in the same person; often, they exist simultaneously. Aren't we kind and nasty sometimes? Aren't we scattered and concentrated? We just manifest one quality or the other from moment to moment.

We're so vast, so complicated, so unfathomable. It seems a shame to live on just the one level of ourselves—intellect, emotions, body urges, whatever—that happens to be dominant. Each one of us is such a wealth of traits and potentials, how can we not bring great wisdom to every situation we encounter if we have access to all of our levels? Don't we all need the capacity to react at both ends of any continuum in order to respond to the complex situations of our lives in this perplexing world? Shouldn't we sometimes allow ourselves to be moved by the wondrous visions of our teachers and friends, and other times can't we understand that it is our charge to be firm, to hold the line? I think this may well be the art of living: mustering the discipline to focus attention in a one-pointed way but developing the wisdom that knows when to step back and allow many levels of ourselves to bubble up in life situations. Carl Jung is supposed to have observed that consistency is the mark of mediocrity. I couldn't agree more. Why be a one-trick pony when there are so many horses in the stable to be ridden?

In order to assure ourselves of the emotional support we all need, we must take a close look at our habit patterns and decide whether we can nourish ourselves or are overly harsh with ourselves like disapproving parents. These attitudes apply in the realms of sexuality, physical comfort, creativity, and respect for our own emotional needs. This investigation requires us to think independently and imaginatively. It is very important to become aware of our attitudes and fears and to question those that interfere with the satisfaction of our emotional needs. This means that everything—our thoughts, feelings, emotions, and actions—is deserving of study. There's no good and bad, holy and profane, from the standpoint of learning to see what we need in our lives to feel nourished and whole and how we behave when we are deprived of this nourishment. Everything in life can be our teacher if we can use the information to study ourselves, our own tendencies, our points of view, our habit patterns. We then understand that it's not a matter of perfecting ourselves, correcting our faults. It's more a matter of seeing them and taking them into account in the situations in which they arise.

Often when we begin to notice the incongruity between our habits that have gone unquestioned for years (like scrubbing the floors every weekend) and our real values (like honoring a need for unstructured time alone), we realize that being under a lot of stress or in a lot of pain makes the sustenance in our lives more important than ever before. We all need nurturing and pleasure—even more so if we are suffering. Study after study has shown that there is a biochemical concomitant of pleasure and self-nurturing that is often powerful enough to reverse the course of a serious disease.

I believe that even with full participation in today's stressful world, you can find a deeply satisfying and sane way to live if you are willing to take your own needs and yearnings seriously enough to use them as a touchstone for creating the kind of life that broadens and delights you. When, through meditation and the study of your behavior and motivations, you come to value all the different parts of yourself, you are inclined toward nurturing yourself as a matter of course. If you can learn to appreciate yourself as you are, to notice your good intentions and wholehearted efforts, you will find it a joy to care for yourself as tenderly as you would for someone else whom you love.

It would be wise to cultivate the attitude of feeling as if you have all the time in the world to acquaint yourself with how the various aspects of yourself clamor for your attention at any given moment. You respect your inclinations. You sleep, play, work, and relax in turn, as you are disposed and as your commitments to other people and projects allow. If you choose to forgo play or your social life for a while to complete a project that is important to you in some way (as I did to write this book), you understand that you made the decision according to what you value most highly. That way, you are less inclined to fall into "victim" mode, feeling oppressed by an outside force. You can tell you are being nurtured when you are relaxed and unhurried, even in the midst of hectic activity. You know that you are taking the proper care of yourself when you are disposed to be generous to yourself and others and when you have a sense that life—even with its pains, sorrows, and disappointments—is basically worth living.

PERSONAL KOANS

Most of us find it very difficult to penetrate past our ordinary habit patterns into The One Who Is Not Busy, the deep well of creativity within all of us from which we can avail ourselves of all our buried resources. We need access to this intuitive wisdom in order to inform the decisions we make in our daily lives. Some people do formal meditation for years without being able to generalize the insights they have on their cushions in the quiet of their early mornings to the rush and tumble of their afternoons. Other people turn to psychotherapists to widen the arenas of their struggles and multiply their choices. Still they come up against huge areas of themselves that therapy might not have touched because the territory is too deep, too primal, beyond words or concepts.

A method I have found very useful for this kind of inquiry is that of formulating a question that touches on the area of my life that perplexes me. Then I keep asking myself the question at all times of the day, setting it before myself in all kinds of circumstances. This type of focused concentration on my question pulls up a response from a part of myself that wasn't available to me when I started asking the question. This is a personal, modern version of a respected, time-honored method used in various schools of Zen for centuries: the practice of koan study.

Koans have been used since ancient times as adjuncts to meditation practice to undermine habitual perception by interrupting the internal dialogue that maintains it. So framing a koan, a question that relates to your life, and then asking it of yourself throughout your day is very much a mindfulness practice, with the same intention. Koans provide a point to which you can return during any state of mind or physical activity. Just coming back to a koan repeatedly throughout your day during many different activities cuts through the fast-flowing stream of thoughts for just a moment and allows you to plant your pole in the rushing river, to establish your banner of truth in the midst of the onslaught of conflicting ideas.

I first became aware of the enormous power of consciously practicing with a koan when I lived at Green Gulch Farm, a Zen farming community in Marin County, California, and wanted to quit smoking cigarettes. It was extremely inconvenient to be a smoker in a meditation community, a place where smoking not only was socially unacceptable but was seen as tantamount to being so oblivious to your mental and physical health as to be virtually comatose. (This was the midseventies, so we were ahead of our time in our intolerance of smokers' rights.) Of course, no physical supports like ashtrays or matches were available in public areas, so in addition to fending off the disapproving glances of all my fellow Zen students, I had to carry around my own ashtray and matches as well as my cigarettes.

Although I had tried many times over the years to give up smoking, I had never succeeded for more than a few weeks. By the time I came to Green Gulch, I had pretty much accepted myself as a hopeless, if hapless, addict. But now my smoking had resurfaced as an issue at Green Gulch because I had to wonder why I, a person with a low tolerance for protracted aggravation, was still driven to smoke in such a hostile environment.

The reason I decided to frame this relatively pedestrian problem as a koan was that Richard Baker, my Zen teacher, had exhorted me constantly and sternly to stop complaining about my shortcomings and start seeing them as opportunities to study myself and my patterns of mind. Stopping smoking struck me as an ideal subject for study because it was a little snippet, a small unit, of my behavior that I could get my novice's mind around, as opposed to some deep-seated conflict that would have to be dredged from the depths of my psyche. So I asked the question, Why is smoking so important to me?

I set about studying this question by noticing everything I could about my desire to smoke and the act of smoking: What was I thinking just before I reached for a cigarette? While I was lighting up? What was my experience during the first drag? When I put the cigarette down in the ashtray? When I picked it up again? When I ground it out? Since I had to carry around all the apparatus and plan my smokes during the natural breaks in the highly structured Green Gulch day, smoking had already often seemed to me like the organizing principle of my life. Now it became much worse because even more of my attention was devoted to smoking than before. Not only did I have to perform all the operations of smoking, I had to be conscious of them as well. Though I didn't yet realize it, in that very focus of consciousness lies much of the tremendous power of a koan to permeate the usual habit patterns of our minds. In *Meditating with Koans,* J. C. Cleary brings us the eleventh-century Zen teacher Wuzu Kayan's admonition: "Putting a koan in contact with your roiling mind is like putting a ladleful of cold water into a pot of boiling water."

Well, I reached past my roiling mind to notice every possible thing about my smoking. Before I began this koan practice, my expectation was that I would quit smoking because I was really experiencing, for the first time without flinching away, how obnoxious a habit it was in its many manifestations: carrying all that gear around, having to separate myself from other people, being aware of their overweening disapproval whenever they happened to spot me off in the corner puffing away, waiting longingly for the breaks in the day when I could indulge myself, and now, since I was paying attention, I could actually feel the toxic smoke being sucked down into my lungs. It seemed quite reasonable to expect this multifaceted vexation to end my attachment to smoking.

But it didn't seem to be going in that direction at all. Instead, after five days of this strenuous observation, I realized how much smoking meant to me and that I couldn't possibly live without it. It seemed like a lifesaver! I saw that my energy and intention weren't equal to the requirements of my demanding life in the Zen community. I needed the little spaces smoking created in my day to relax, to withdraw from other people, to totally space out and, for the two or three minutes it took to smoke a cigarette, not be responsible for anything, even my thoughts. It actually panicked me to think of my life without those precious moments when I inhaled smoke down into my lungs and exhaled it out into the air, those languorous, sensuous moments when my life belonged to no one but me.

Observing this, I thought to myself, This whole dream of giving up smoking is hopeless. I will never be able to give it up as long as I live. It wasn't that I had taken up the koan in order to quit smoking. In accordance with the usual procedures for embarking on koan study, I had just asked my question—Why am I so attached to smoking?—and made my observations. But nevertheless, I had hoped that if I thoroughly registered my suffering each moment I was causing it, certainly I would want to stop.

What I didn't realize was how koans work in the mind. I now believe they set up an unconscious process that reverberates through the mind and resonates in every corner. In Michael Wenger's book of modern koans *33 Fingers,* Richard Baker tells a story that illustrates how koans work subterraneously. In the koan Wenger calls "The Brown Telephone," Baker said, "I dreamt I was trying to solve a problem. A brown phone kept ringing in the background, distracting me. Finally, annoyed, I picked it up and the voice on the other end told me the answer to the problem."

As Thomas Cleary puts it in *No Barrier: Unlocking the Zen Koan,* koans foster the ability to engage an extra dimension of attention at will. But even more important, the mind is developed in the very process of calling koans to attention. When you develop the capacity to practice a koan in the course of all activities, you develop a consciousness that can continue its uninterrupted observation regardless of whether there is calm or disturbance in your thoughts or surroundings. "The very act of bringing up a koan at that time asserts the original freedom and independence of the mind. The fortitude of heart this produces cannot be duplicated by fabricated meditation procedures. When thus empowered, the mind is not obstructed by ordinary affairs but can manage them with freedom of choice."

Despite my noticing how hopelessly attached and addicted I was to smoking, in another few days, I had spontaneously quit with no effort beyond the conscious observation of my smoking. It seemed like a miracle to me. I had always believed abstractly in the power of the unconscious mind, but now, directly observing its mysterious workings, I was deeply moved. What I think happened during my koan study was that I gradually started to inhabit the "languorous, sensuous moments," once entirely filled by smoking, with my observations, my presence. I brought a little energy into those small gaps in awareness, and it enlivened them. I didn't do it intentionally. It just happened in the process of the koan study. This was my first koan, and I was tremendously impressed with the power of one-pointed mind to penetrate and diffuse itself over the entire consciousness with no conscious direction from me! Just as Thomas Cleary so eloquently put it.

So I fell in love with koans that first time out and have since used them in many different guises and situations. I have also recommended their use to friends and students. I think personal koans help tremendously to penetrate the tired, habitual way we look at our lives and activities. They are a way to bring our meditation into our everyday lives. By framing a habit of mind or a troubling problem as a question or a point of focus that we come back to in all mental states during all kinds of activities, we reach past our usual ways of thinking about these things. It's also important that we widen our screen in a curious, exploratory way, not necessarily looking for immediate answers or results. The framing of the question ought to reflect an attitude of inquiry; we're positing a frame of reference from which to watch a certain aspect of our reality, as I did with smoking. What seems crucial to me is the proper framing and reframing of a question so that it excites curiosity and invites nonjudgmental exploration. Our everyday life questions can be made into a tool that penetrates our conditioned habits in the same way that a drill bores through wood.

I have found over the years that the most useful koans for me have been the questions that arose from my concerns about the particular ways I function in everyday life: my relationships, my ability to work, my sense of connection with my activity. The most persistent, most troubling problem I had as a young person was the sense that there was some kind of invisible shield that separated me from my experience. As a teenager, I noticed that when I was doing something, I always felt that I wasn't fully engaged, that there were huge parts of me that weren't available for my life. It was very frustrating to feel perpetually split up, inattentive, preoccupied. I attributed it to the fact that my life in a midwestern suburb was boring. Nothing interesting or exciting ever happened to me. I hoped that maybe if something exciting did happen someday—my overheated imagination concocted scenarios constantly—I would be amazed enough to give it all my attention, open-eyed. But I also feared that maybe nothing would command that much respect from my meandering, ill-mannered brain.

As a young woman, I developed some strategies to deal with this feeling of separation. I noted the unusual alertness roused in my normally distracted mind whenever I fell in love. Instead of its usual endless and thoughtless chatter, once it was aroused by hormonal stimulation, my consciousness seemed riveted to one focus: the object of my desire. I was awakened from a kind of slumber by love. So my first theory in penetrating my invisible shield was that only being in love could melt it away. Once aroused to love, I could give my full attention to things. This worked very well for short periods of time. I would meet someone totally engaging, fall in love, and regard him and everything else with vivid attention. My invisible shield would evaporate from sheer heat. I was fully alive and happy. But eventually the shield would return, and my inevitable haze would overcome my love. I just couldn't stay in love uncritically, unanxiously, unconditionally, long enough to create a permanent shift in the workings of my roiling mind.

My next strategy was based on the notion that since this invisible shield was a defect of attention and presence, I might be able to penetrate it if I could set up my life so that I rarely did anything that I didn't totally love doing. I thought maybe I could completely bury my shield in good works that I believe in, shoulder to shoulder with other committed people. I became part of a political group that was working to stop the Vietnam War. However, after a short but passionate time full of meetings and demonstrations and doctrinal arguments, the gap was back. Rather than join me to my activity, my political work caused me to feel angry and separated from most of the world. My idealism and lack of experience in the world allowed me to project my anger and isolation on groups of people outside my trusted circle of friends. I began dividing the world very simplistically into the exploiters and the exploited. I remember jerking my dog away when a policeman, a storm trooper lackey of the military-industrial complex, tried to pet him.

This kind of alienation based on doctrine was extremely painful to me. It's not in my nature to embrace abstract ideals to the exclusion of actual human beings. So despite the kind of camaraderie I enjoyed with my fellow revolutionaries, my devotion to a just cause backfired on me, swelling the chasm of my loneliness to a point where it was nearly unendurable. I thought of suicide. If I couldn't somehow fully inhabit my life, regardless of what the specifics of that life were, then it didn't seem worth living. At the time, I complained that I hadn't found the right lover or the right line of work yet, that if I could just do one or both of those things, I would be fulfilled. Secretly I was terrified that it would never happen.

When I came to the San Francisco Zen Center, my teacher Richard Baker gave me an opportunity to study my problem in a way I never had before. He suggested I look into the habit patterns of my thoughts to find my invisible shield, specifically my habit of waiting for something to happen to me that deserved my full attention. He told me, "Look into your waiting." I tried to follow his advice, but my habit of waiting for some worthy event to occur was so much a part of me that at first, I couldn't even see it; it was like my own nose. But visibility is one of the useful attributes of a personal koan; it puts something out there in front of you to look at. Since I was very determined to "look into my waiting," I had to find where in my thoughts or attitudes my waiting was.

It took a lot of effort and time before I found my invisible shield at last in particular thoughts I had that separated me from what I was doing, like hurrying through my laundry and cleaning chores on my day off from work so that I could "enjoy" myself when they were done. I would rush through them as fast as I could, thinking of and looking forward to that moment when my "real life" would start. But when I finished my chores and my "real life" arrived, pregnant with possibility, the moment I had been waiting for . . . there was nothing really spectacular to do, no superhuman lover who would never disappoint me, no transporting activity worthy of my great talents. There was just . . . more boring life.

It took many days off to locate the life that was being squandered in the waiting. To find the places I didn't inhabit—like the spaces I had filled by inhaling smoke from a cigarette—the particular thoughts by which I didn't inhabit them, and then to start to inhabit them, consciously and fervently, with my attention. To start to be alive for the laundry, conscious during the dish washing, aware of my body as I walked to the store, and—this was big—looking into another person's face and seeing that person, not some dream I was dreaming that I put between us, the invisible shield settling onto a real person's features.

In light of what may seem to be a koan's enormous potential to plunge past our mundane chatter into our silent depths, it would seem very important to frame the perfect question. But I have found this is not necessarily so. The koan seems to have a self-correcting mechanism. Just starting with a sincere and earnest question about your life may be quite enough if you will come back to that question again and again during your day. Then the question itself will change and evolve into another one, which you will again repeat and bring yourself to in the course of your daily activity. Then your question will change again with your evolving awareness of its scope.

Friends and students have shared their own personal koans with me, and I think sharing some of them with you may help you formulate your own question. After you have a question, then you can watch what seems to be its independent evolution as it permeates your consciousness. One woman I know with a demanding job, an estranged husband, and three teenagers complained constantly over the years that she was giving of herself all the time and not getting much back in the way of psychological support. When I suggested formulating her concern into a question, she immediately responded with, "Where do I begin, and where do I end?"

Just a few weeks after starting to practice with that question, she was amazed at what she had learned about herself. "What a sponge for other people's feelings I am!" she exclaimed. "I'm pulled off my own agenda all the time by other people's immediate needs. I always value theirs higher than my own." She said she felt that she was "hyperopen," unable to set limits on her own availability. She did, however, begin to feel the stirrings of a choice, where she might draw the line if she were going to start drawing a line. That both scared and thrilled her. So her first question was leading her into her deep beliefs about the importance of meeting other people's expectations and what she thought might be the consequences of considering her own needs on a par with those of others.

A good example of how the first question we formulate evolves into other, deeper questions came from a friend who missed a lover in her life and wondered whether she distanced herself from men in some unconscious way. Her first question was, "How would it feel to be loved?" In just a few days, that became "How would it feel to love?" In another few weeks, she was asking herself, "How do I love?" As she called her question up during the course of her day, her mind was drawn to emphasize first one word, then another. The subject had been stale for her for years; even her longing and sadness had eventually turned into numbness. Now she felt lively, eagerly attuned to how she connected with people, her curiosity about her own behavior aroused by her question. She found it especially fascinating to notice all the details of other people's appreciation of her: whether she noticed compliments when she got them, whether they were enough for her, how appreciation made her feel anytime it arose.

She also reported a "side effect": since posing the question about her loneliness, she had started feeling something very different, very dynamic, about it. Studying her behavior and other people's responses to her seemed in themselves to ease her loneliness! Just becoming aware of her interactions seemed to make her feel more connected. She realized that her social relationships had been more reflexive than actual encounters with other human beings. In a few weeks, she had located her distancing mechanism.

A charming, dapper man I know well had his completely absorbing social life forever changed by a tragic car accident that disabled him. Three years after the accident forced him into early retirement, he was restless, lonely, and frustrated. Encounters with former coworkers and old friends, frequent at first but now rare, only upset him. The gap between their active lives and what his had become was too stark for him to continue those old relationships. He desperately needed new companions, new ways to pursue his interests. Everyone around him tried to be helpful, making suggestions about how he might connect with new people, but he always found reasons why the suggested approaches wouldn't work. He even told me once that he wasn't befriending the people in his support group because he didn't want to hang out with "handicapped people." I was struck with what self-loathing must be behind that statement. After he related to me a couple of incidents that demonstrated how impossible it was for him to meet suitable people, I suggested he work with the question "What do I do that separates me from people?"

He took up the question with his usual dedication and intelligence. I didn't hear from him for a month. When I did see him, he told me frankly that he had experienced tremendous despair as a result of working with this question. He shocked me by telling me that in the course of this inquiry, he had spontaneously returned to the scene of his accident for the first time in many years. He had always avoided the place in his travels around town. As he sat there in his car, he was overwhelmed by grief and sorrow for the life that had been destroyed at that very spot. He understood that a part of him would never get over mourning for his old life.

As he continued to work with his koan, he began to understand that his knee-jerk rejection of other people struggling with pain was a projection of his own perceived unattractiveness. He just couldn't imagine being of value or interest to anyone else in his current condition. Seeing that the thoughts that kept him separate from others were his own both devastated and enlivened him. Although he hated to think he saw himself and other disabled people as unworthy, he now also felt free to get beyond an unconscious prejudice that was stymieing his social life.

A woman very active in local politics developed such severe tendinitis in her arms that she was gradually forced to curtail her work hours at the computer to the point where she lost her job as a highly paid pollster. Although she looked completely normal, and her network of friends had not diminished at all, she was utterly panicked about her inability to heal. She had been to every kind of physical therapist, medical practitioner, and body worker without improving, or even maintaining, her health. She noticed the subtle but steady loss of function from week to week, and by the time she confided in me, she was hysterical with worry. Since she couldn't imagine how she was damaging herself, she couldn't halt her relentless degeneration. I recommended that she begin at once to meditate on the sensations of her own body in order to discover any conflict she might be setting up between her will and her body's inclinations. Her question became "What would it be like to live in my body?"

She surprised me in the following days with her accounts of just how disconnected she had been, not only from her body itself but from her whole physical environment. She regaled me with the new appreciation she had for the things around her: flowers, trees, even the architecture of San Francisco. "I can't believe how beautiful this city is!" she told me. I said, "You mean you never noticed the Victorians, the bay, the fog sweeping down over the hills before?" She shook her head, chagrined. She had lived her entire life in her head, preoccupied with her thoughts, emotions, and opinions, oblivious to her surroundings. In a few weeks, her question had changed into "What does it feel like to be a body?"

Bright and observant, she had almost no trouble locating the ideas she had that interfered with her physical healing. She put tremendous strain on her body when she forced it to obey her notions of what her activity level should be. Even out of work, she continued her rounds of social activities and vigorous exercise, which were inappropriate for her body. At first, it seemed foreign to her to take her body's point of view, especially since rest was what it craved, but soon she was reveling in it, delighted with her expanding awareness of the world, both inside and out. In a few months, her degeneration had stopped (to her doctor's amazement). Nearly a year later, she had gained so much strength and stamina she began looking for new work—a quest she undertook firmly planted in a body she had come to love and respect.

Formulating a Personal Koan

1. Practice formulating a concise question that reflects the primary issue in your life right now. It may be that you can't get a handle on the main issue right away, that you feel some vague dissatisfaction but don't know how to frame a specific question about it. Just starting to think about what your question might be will help you penetrate to your real concern. You might start with something very general like "What is my suffering?" Then your practice of putting this question before yourself and your observation of what comes up for you when you ask it will gradually sculpt the question into something very personal and specific.

2. Repeat your koan (a) when you brush your teeth, (b) as you begin each meal, (c) whenever you rise to take a walk, (d) before you fall asleep.

It is certainly true that when we frame our problems as questions, our ultimate hope is to change our circumstances. Once asked, however, the question itself stimulates curiosity and a desire for information about the current situation that become stronger than the need to change it. Framing problems as questions really helps to dispel the attachment to results that our minds always bring to every activity they take up. Although the wish to change our circumstances may be what initially motivates us to formulate the problems of our everyday lives into a koan—we want things to run more smoothly, we want to achieve a goal—the process of asking questions, of setting our koan before us in many situations again and again, circumvents the tendency to measure all our observations in terms of the end product. I think what koans do is shift our attention to what is rather than what we wish it to be. Michael Wenger remarks in *33 Fingers: A Collection of Modern American Koans:*

> Our ordinary life situations and encounters afford us the opportunity to recognize our boundless essential nature seen through the lens of the most ordinary events. . . . A problem

can be a treasure if we know how to practice with it. At that time a problem is not necessarily something to be solved, but a valuable tool to open the body-mind in a way that gives access to our complete undivided "big self."

It is this kind of awareness of our depths and our ability to respond to the life that arises for us moment by moment right under our feet that makes our lives compelling and vital, reflective of our deepest yearnings and satisfactions.

SOURCES AND CREDITS

❧ ❧

Wonderful works, all.

Aitken, Robert. *The Mind of Clover*. San Francisco: North Point Press, 1984.

Anderson, Reb. "Sitting in the Heart of Suffering: Where the Clouds Crop Up." *The Windbell* (magazine published periodically by the San Francisco Zen Center) 19, no. 1 (Summer 1985).

Barrows, Anita. "The Light of Outrage." In *Buddhist Women on the Edge*, edited by Marianne Dresser. Berkeley, Calif.: North Atlantic Books, 1996.

Beck, Joko. *Everyday Zen*. San Francisco: Harper & Row, 1989.

Cleary, J. C. *Meditating with Koans*. Berkeley, Calif.: Asian Humanities Press, 1992.

Cleary, Thomas. *No Barrier: Unlocking the Zen Koan*. New York: Bantam, 1993.

Cleary, Thomas, and J. C. Cleary, trans. *The Blue Cliff Record*. Vol. 1. Boston: Shambhala Publications, 1977.

Epstein, Mark. *Thoughts without a Thinker*. New York: Basic Books, 1995.

Friedman, Lenore, and Susan Moon, eds. *Being Bodies*. Boston: Shambhala Publications, 1997.

Guenther, Herbert. *Philosophy and Psychology in the Abhidharma*. Boston: Shambhala Publications, 1976.

Hanh, Thich Nhat. *The Miracle of Mindfulness: A Manual of Meditation*. Boston: Beacon Press, 1976.

Kabat-Zinn, Jon. *Full Catastrophe Living*. New York: Delta, 1990.

Katagiri, Dainin. "True Heart: Raising the Banner of Truth." *The Windbell* 19, no. 1 (Summer 1985).

Kornfield, Jack. *A Path with Heart*. New York: Bantam, 1993.

Ornish, Dean. "Changing Life Habits." In *Healing and the Mind*, edited by Bill Moyers. New York: Doubleday, 1995.

Siegel, Bernie, M.D. *Love, Medicine and Miracles*. New York: Harper & Row, 1986.

Suzuki, Shunryu. *Zen Mind, Beginner's Mind*. New York: Weatherhill, 1970, 1986.

Tanahashi, Kazuaki, ed. *Moon in a Dewdrop: Writings of Zen Master Dogen*. New York: North Point Press, 1985.

Tanahashi, Kazuaki, and David Schneider, eds. *Essential Zen*. Edison, N.J.: Castle Books, 1996.

Trungpa Rinpoche, Chögyam. *Cutting through Spiritual Materialism*. Boston: Shambhala Publications, 1973.

———. *Shambhala: The Sacred Path of the Warrior*. Boston: Shambhala Publications, 1984.

Wenger, Michael. *33 Fingers: A Collection of Modern American Koans*. San Francisco: Clear Glass Publishing, 1994.

HIPBONE PRODUCTIONS

255 LAGUNA STREET, SAN FRANCISCO, CA 94102

ORDER FORM

Living with Arthritis: Self-Help
Morning Workout with Darlene Cohen
VIDEOTAPE
(Includes instructional booklet)   _____ copies @ $30.00 _____

BOOKLET without videotape   _____ copies @ $ 4.00 _____

Arthritis: Stop Suffering, Start Moving—Everyday
Exercises for Body and Mind
Paperback book by Darlene Cohen   _____ copies @ $14.95 _____

AUDIOTAPES

TWO MEDITATIONS
Side 1: On Release of Pain
Side 2: Body and Breath   _____ copies @ $10.00 _____

MEDITATION ON MOVEMENT
Side 1: Body Awareness
Side 2: Relational Movement   _____ copies @ $10.00 _____

California residents: $8\frac{1}{2}$% tax   _____

Postage and handling (USA: multiply order by 15%;
outside USA: multiply order by 20%)   _____

                                        TOTAL: _____

Enclose check or money order to:
HIPBONE PRODUCTIONS

BE SURE TO INCLUDE YOUR ADDRESS:

Name: _____

Address: _____

          _____

THANK YOU FOR YOUR ORDER!